Diagnosis: CANCER

Diagnosis: CANCER

How does cancer arise?
How can it be treated?
A hypothesis and a therapy
which promise success

Waltraut Fryda

Copyright © 2006 by Waltraut Fryda.

Library of Congress Control Number: 2005908927
ISBN: Hardcover   1-59926-898-1
               Softcover   1-59926-897-3

All rights reserved. No part of this book may be reproduced or transmitted in any form or by any means, electronic or mechanical, including photocopying, recording, or by any information storage and retrieval system, without permission in writing from the copyright owner.

This book was printed in the United States of America.

To order additional copies of this book, contact:
Xlibris Corporation
1-888-795-4274
www.Xlibris.com
Orders@Xlibris.com
31145

CONTENTS

Foreword 13

Introduction 15
    Biology is today's dominant science. A brief history of the development of biology. The cell as building block of life. Biology and medicine are not "exact" sciences. The hypothesis on the origins of cancer and the therapy introduced in this book are not outside conventional medicine, they are not alternative. Both hypothesis and therapy are founded on a consistent, natural basis.

Life Is Permanently Endangered 20
    Life is an open-ended system, quite unlike thermodynamic equilibrium. The fundamental building block is the cell. Life is continuously exposed to manifold threats, from microorganisms to wrong nutrition, from physical to psychological influences. The fact of survival makes it possible to establish strategies that have developed through evolution. Nevertheless, illnesses arise, and premature death occurs. Cancer is on the increase, very often leading to death.

What Is Cancer? 22
    A brief definition. Benign and malignant cell changes. Which characteristics distinguish a cancer cell from a normal cell? Various manifestations of cancer. Known risk factors.

Brief Summary on the Topic of Cancer 24
    The molecular aspect. The classical dogma on the formation of cancer. Tumor-suppressor genes versus oncogenes. Doubts over the classical dogma arising from confusing, partly contradictory findings in tumor cells. Chaos in the chromosomes and yet no disintegration of structure and function of the cancer cell.

The Hypothesis on the Origin of Cancer 26
    Adrenaline deficiency as cause for the onset of cancer. Exhaustion of the chromaffin system through stress over a long period of time. Impaired acid—alkali balance. Weakening of the immune defense. Impairment of the interaction between adrenaline and insulin. Glycogen overload and oxygen deficiency in cells. Anaerobic, i.e., restricted, cell metabolism as emergency measure.

The Hormone Adrenaline 30
    Its most important functions.

Sugar Metabolism 31
Adrenaline, the important antagonist to insulin.

Oxygen Supply 31
The effect of adrenaline and noradrenaline on blood vessels.

Metabolism in Case of Insufficient Oxygen 32
Aerobic and anaerobic metabolism. Evolutionary relationship of prokaryonts and eukaryonts. Flexibility in the metabolism of eukaryonts. Metabolism of fermentation. The universal ATP (adenosine triphosphate) energy household. Glycogen mast of the cell. Glycolysis in muscle cells and erythrocytes. The stress hormone adrenaline also stimulates the defense mechanisms.

The Immune System 35
Congenital and adaptive immunity. Cellular and humoral immune response. Pathogens and antigens. Granulocytes, macrophages, B cells, and T cells. Antibodies. Failure of immune defense in the presence of malignant cells.

Insulin Effect 39
Adrenaline deficiency results in hyperinsulinism. Transmutation of genes into oncogenes. Transition to carcinogenesis. Damage of lysosomes. Insulin and cancer growth. Diabetic metabolism and tumors.

Substitute Reactions in Case of Adrenaline Deficiency 42
Substitute reactions taking over upon failure of adrenaline production that lead to the development of compensatory effects. The various hormones, which in their overproduction, lead to damaging side effects within the organism.

    Thyroid Hormones 43

    Adrenal Cortical Hormones 43

    Growth Hormone STH 44

    Glucagon 44

    Summary of Substitute Reactions 45

Paraneoplastic Hormone Changes 46
Spread of symptoms of a tumor or its metastases on a humoral path. ACTH. Growth hormone. Thyrotropin. Calcitonin. Follicle-stimulating hormone. Luteinising hormone. The ectopic formation of erythropoietin, hypoglycemia, and cachexia.

Acid-Alkali Household 48
pH value. Natural interaction between blood-pH value and tissue-pH value. Impaired acid-alkali household of the organism as cause for nearly all chronic diseases. An acid environment of *tissue* adversely affects cell respiration and promotes the formation of the first malignant cell. An increased alkalisation

of the *blood* endangers the stability of many vital hormones, in particular that of adrenaline.

Stress 51

Stress and stressor. Hyperstress and hypostress. Eustress and distress. Stress is necessary, but can be damaging—an equilibrium phenomenon. Varying models. The three-phase general adaptation syndrome (Selye syndrome). The exhaustion phase as axis of the cancer-formation hypothesis. Physical and psychological stressors. Oxidative stress. The particular stress situation of cancer patients.

Is There a "Typical Cancer Personality"? 56

A discussion of personality characteristics (but not hereditary traits). The existence of choleric, melancholic, phlegmatic, and sanguine personalities was acknowledged in ancient times. Differentiation between two types of fear reaction: vagotonic and sympathicotonic. A cancer patient has a vagotonic personality. Stress-management strategies are all important.

Phases of Cancer Formation 59

The varied causes of a cancer illness build up over many years. Cancer patients and their "blank sheet" of ailments. The changes in the immune situation over many years allow recognition of four phases of cancer formation: normergy, allergy, hypergy, anergy.

The Therapy 62

The Diet 62

Detoxification of the intestines with a cancer-hostile diet.

Acid-Alkali Ratio 65

Depriving the tumor of its acid environment. Administration of dextrorotatory lactic acid for the deacidifaction of tissues. The "changeover reaction". Dextrorotatory lactic acid stimulates adrenaline production. At the same time, it neutralizes the toxic levorotatory lactic acid into a racemic form.

Restitution of Adrenaline Production 66

Stimulating the body's own hormone production by means of suitable cell and organ preparations, as administration of adrenaline injections is counterproductive.

Enzymes, Vitamins 67

Prescription of a combination of digestion enzymes to facilitate the destruction of tumor particles. Additional supply of vitamins A, B, and C.

Sex Hormones 68

Examining the administration of opposite-sex hormones for sex-hormone-related tumors. Replacement of oestrogen and progesterone for female patients. No administration of sex hormones for tumors with corresponding receptors.

Concluding Observations to the Therapy 68
Little stress for the patient. The history of the cancer illness from its origin becomes the focal point. Motive and objective of treatment are always clear: stimulation of adrenaline production and, thus, a normalisation of the cell metabolism.

Outlook 69
Greater emphasis on the formation of the cancer and less on the cancer cell itself. Further tasks arising from such an approach: extensive, analogous laboratory tests to monitor progress of the therapy. Establishing measurement parameters for long-term studies on the development of cancer.

Is It Possible to Protect Oneself Against Cancer? 71
Social impositions on individuals, which are in collision with our genetic makeup for dealing with stress. Unavoidable social and cultural circumstances often trigger the formation of cancer. Progress through understanding of these correlations.

A Selection of Case Histories of Cured Patients 74

Glossary 77

References 81

Index 83

Dedicated in memory of my sons,
Thomas and Axel

He who knows the goal can decide.
He who decides finds peace.
He who finds peace is secure.
He who is secure can reflect.
He who reflects can improve.

—Confucius

Foreword

In the spring of 2003, it was decided to thoroughly overhaul my book on the origins of cancer, which was first published in 1984. Although practical experience with the therapy has increased in the meantime to an inestimable degree, the core itself of the hypothesis on the origins of cancer has remained unchanged, and interest in this therapy has continued to remain unabated; in fact, it continues to increase. The decision for a new edition after nineteen years is easily understood, considering, in my view, the traumatic effect this immense topic has on people. Furthermore, I am more than ever convinced that I have shown a right way, which I myself have followed. The patients whom I have been able to help over all these years are my yardstick for this.

To start off, this new edition was completely restructured on the one hand to facilitate reading for the lay public and on the other hand to make available to a broader interested readership and more in-depth details. These are not always strictly subject related but at times also establish historic or other connections. I trust that this has been achieved with the choice of two different-type fonts in the main text. The smaller print can initially be read in a more casual manner without losing the core connection. Furthermore, a more extensive glossary has been added, which endeavors to explain the meaning of topical expressions, the inclusion of which is unavoidable. Lay readers and doctors will no doubt use this to varying degrees—one perhaps more, the other less.

I consider that the individual subtopics have been highlighted more clearly, resulting in a clearer structure. I hope that this too will promote the understanding of a sometimes rather complicated subject matter.

Furthermore, new main focal points have been created, as becomes clear from the chapters dealing with the immune system, the acid-alkali household, stress, and in particular the therapy. And finally, I hope the reader will discover new thought processes and completely new chapters, such as "Is there a 'typical cancer personality'?" or "Is it possible to protect oneself against cancer?"

Introduction

This new edition (2003) coincides with the fiftieth anniversary of the revolutionary discovery of the double-helix structure of the genetic material DNA (deoxyribonucleic acid), by Crick and Watson.[1] Enormous progress has been made during these fifty years, especially in molecular biology, to the general benefit of subordinate disciplines such as medicine. Whereas in the beginning, the great discoveries of modern physics and chemistry fundamentally changed our views of the world; nowadays the results of biological research hold our attention, not the least because they are capable of moving us emotionally more than new theories, such as superstring theories or parallel universes, however imposing these may be. During the first half of the twentieth century, physics was clearly the leading science; it can now be argued that during the second half biology has taken over its place and that this dominance is on the increase. Modern physics and chemistry have radically changed our worldview; modern biology is now changing our view on human beings.

What is life? How did it start? How does our organism function? And furthermore, what is spirit? Is there a soul? How is our brain organized? What is consciousness and free will? These are all questions which directly affect us all, and answers to these are relevant for us. Sooner rather than later, they will fundamentally shake up our social and ethical/moral values. Human medicine is particularly affected by this, when one considers the debates on cloning, preimplantation selection of embryos, stem-cell extraction, active euthanasia, gene therapy, definition of guilt in penal legislation in line with new findings in brain research—these are only a few examples which make daily headlines in the media. Great expectations are placed on innovative advances in the fight against various illnesses, which cannot be cured as yet, whether these are infectious diseases, hereditary diseases, or cancer.

Medicine gained enormous ground from the vast advances in cytology (scientific research of cells), and yet the prevailing treatment methods for cancer, which the layman understands to be a malignant rampaging of cells, are the so-called primary therapies: i.e., operation, radiation, and chemotherapy. Do such procedures not have a "rather mechanical" sound? Man is often considered like a machine that can be repaired and treated accordingly. This seems to be all the more absurd if one considers that a human—and animal—organism, even a single-celled organism, by far exceeds every man-made device, including the most sophisticated computer or the smallest nanomachines in complexity, originality, elegance, or completeness. Of course, evolution spanned millions of years; measured against this, the time invested by modern science in research is minute. We are just at the beginning of understanding the development processes and the manifold characteristics of living things.

> The oldest fossils—cyanobacteria, microorganisms with prokaryotic cell structure, which perform photosynthesis, releasing oxygen—are approximately 3.5 billion years old. It took nearly two billion years until the first true cells with a nucleus (eukaryotes) appeared, from which we all derive.[2]

> The beginnings of the scientific revolution, introduced with the Copernican turning point, date back more than five hundred years. Up to the present, this has not been a straight path. What started with the ordering of the world picture[3] and is linked to the names of Copernicus, Galileo, and in particular Descartes and Newton, initially found many approving voices. Although Descartes did not go so far as denying that man has a soul, animals were to him only automatons. Later, Cartesian theory reached its peak with Julien Offray de la Mettrie's *L'homme Machine* (1749). However, opponents appeared, who could not accept mechanical explanations. Vitalism developed in the early seventeenth century, i.e., the belief that "living beings have at their disposal a special life force or substance of life, which is lacking in lifeless matter."[2] Although it was not possible to define this life force, it was decisively affirmed that there was a fundamental difference between lifeless matter and living organisms. Vitalism was finally overtaken by modern genetics and the concept of a genetic program and by Darwinism with its principles of variation and natural selection (Charles Darwin, *Origin of Species*, 1859). Life is a self-organizing process, and the existence of a life force is not required to explain it. Biology is a prime example of reconciliation of two opposing viewpoints, which on their own are insufficient to explain the phenomenon of life: specifically reductionism and holism. Reductionism, according to which complex phenomena of the living world are reduced to their smallest particles, the understanding of which is then considered sufficient to explain higher integration levels of those complex systems, has led to great successes in biology (the cell as unit of all living matter, the universal, molecular structure of DNA, etc.). However, it was unable to explain living matter, either in single-cell form or in higher life-forms. Along the way to ever smaller particles on ever lower levels, something seems to have been lost. The holistic approach (consideration of the whole) on the other hand does not bring us nearer to a solution of the problems.

"The whole is more than the sum total of parts" always sounded a little metaphysical. Today it is known that in a structured system on higher integration levels new characteristics arise, which cannot be derived from the knowledge of the components of lower levels.[2] There is also talk of emerging characteristics (emergence), which is not at all metaphysical. I will return to this important thought later.

It is in no way intended to advance here a simplified method of looking at things; life is highly complex. In particular, there is probably no other system more complex than the live human brain with its approximately one hundred billion neurons, which each has thousands of interlinked connections. It is intended only to emphasize that an understanding of living matter can be achieved, in principle at least.

Returning to the original topic. I felt it was necessary to make this extremely condensed diversion into the history of development of biology, the science of life, in order to clarify to the reader my point of view. The hypothesis on the origins of cancer (carcinogenesis) introduced here does not pursue *alternative* treatment in the modern sense, namely separated from conventional medicine and away from science-based findings. This is not fringe medicine—just the contrary. I endeavor to provide the reader with understanding of biological/medical interrelations. What is the definition of health and illness in human beings, and, in particular geared to the dreaded suffering of cancer, how do malignant tumors arise? Once the development history is understood, the next question is how this understanding can be transformed into a therapy away from normally applied conventional paths. Further to this, it opens the possibility of prevention for all those who may perhaps feel healthy, but whose cancer development has not yet reached the late state of proven tumor formation, because the preconditions for cancer in accordance with the hypothesis under discussion, i.e., the path breakers, are recognisable to the doctor at a relatively early stage. If two principles are seriously considered, namely firstly to recognize at the earliest possible stage the changeover from health (however loose definition may be) to a possible illness and secondly to intervene in the organism with the minimum of corrective, even destructive measures, then the genesis of an illness, cancer in this case, becomes immediately the focal point. Because prevention is always better than treatment.

An important point needs to be emphasized in this context. Biology (and medicine) differs from the so-called exact sciences, such as physics, in particular, in the fact that it relates to matters that are never "the same." Every plant and every animal, even from the same genus, is different; no human being is exactly like the next (disregarding clones for the time being). The truth of this is underlined by the fact that for human beings and animals, *body* and *psyche* go hand in hand. Every individual is exposed to different environmental influences, which do not always lead to the same reactions and behavioral patterns, depending on the existing physical and psychological state, etc. A doctor is of course inclined to recognize "sameness" in patients and to classify, as otherwise he or she would be unable to diagnose an illness. However, often the direct relationship between body and psyche are ignored. Too often, the *objective* diagnosis excludes the *subjective* well-being of the patient; the search for the causes of an illness, its individual development history, and, therefore, the diagnosis, all remain incomplete. This also applies to cancer, where no two patients become ill in the same way. There are always differences, even if they are sometimes small. As is known, cancer expresses itself in varying forms, the common factor of which is, however, always a cell-based degeneration. Although it is not possible to describe it in simple terms, this cell-based degeneration provides the closest "accurate" description of these processes. The onset of degeneration depends on a chain of factors and events, which all can have a multitude of possible causes and focal points: disturbed balances and regulating mechanisms, persistent physical and psychological stress, which are very often very difficult to identify. Medicine is a biological science. Bearing in mind all the above, it could be said that I pursue more a biological method on a consistent, naturalistic basis, but no alternative method in the modern sense of the word.

The hypothesis on the origin of cancer introduced in this book and the therapy derived therefrom differ fundamentally from the three approaches and treatment methods previously stated (namely operation, radiation, chemotherapy), which dominate the field at present. In the beginning and above all else, it is endeavored to establish the development history of a malignant illness in order to draw the necessary conclusions on how the organism can be supported in an appropriate way so that it can cope *on its own* with the malignant illness. This means referral back to the arsenal of nature, which is unique in its effectiveness. The layman should distance himself from the one-dimensional thinking that a cancerous illness "simply erupts" and that the body's own defense mechanisms "quite simply remain inactive in response." Cancer is a systemic illness, and its development history is made up of many layers; whereby, a tumor finally manifests itself as consequence of a series of preceding maldevelopments. In many cases, it may well be justified to attack cancer by means of the above-mentioned primary treatment methods; at the same time, it must be said that one is dealing with later-stage symptoms of a systemic falling ill, the beginning of which goes back quite sometime, completely unnoticed. For example, it is difficult enough to answer after an operation questions as to whether *all* cells of a primary tumor were removed and whether treatment was definitely commenced *prior* to metastasis formation. Even a positively optimistic response to the question does not allow a prognosis of a permanent treatment success to the exclusion of a recurrence of the illness (relapse), because as long as the *general and individual development history* has not been sufficiently researched, advice cannot be given for a change in lifestyle, conducive to the prevention of cancer in future.

In this connection, more recent research[4] is *discouraging*, particularly as regards breast cancer, where sometimes metastases are subsequently discovered without being able to locate the primary cancer focus. This seems to be in contradiction of the prevailing view that a cancerous tumor sends out daughter cells only in an advanced stage.

Even the long-term goal of eventually conquering cancer by immunological means remains vague for as long as the development history of tumor formation, in which a weakening of the immune defense plays an important role, is not understood. It is endeavored to demonstrate this in the hypothesis under discussion.

The presented hypothesis may be incomplete or capable of being refuted in part, but the most important touchstone for it is the treatment success, as is the case for every medical hypothesis. It is important to note at this stage that having been applied in practice for decades, the success of the therapy developed from the hypothesis is on my side. Proof of this will be shown with some selected, anonymous, and summarized patient histories at the end of the book.

Life Is Permanently Endangered

Life is a self-organizing process, a so-called open system far apart from the thermodynamic equilibrium, which requires an external supply of matter and energy (food, respiration) to perform its functions. Its building blocks are cells, all with their own metabolism, from single-celled beings to mammals to human beings.

> The cell is the foundation of all living matter. (A virus is still below this threshold; although it has its own genetic programme in the form of a DNA or RNA molecule, it does not have a metabolism of its own and requires the enzyme mechanism of a host cell for its propagation.) The word "cell" was already used in the first work on cytology: *Micrographia* by *Robert Hooke* from the year 1665. *Theodor Schwann* proved in 1839 that components of animal tissue are nothing less than modified cells, irrespective of how different they seem to be, after *Meyen* and *Schleiden* had already recognized that plants consist exclusively of cells: a pioneering success of reductionism.[2]

In higher life forms, cells are very different both as to structure and function. They are organized in differing cell agglomerations (skin cells, liver cells, brain cells, nerve cells, macrophages, etc.) and interact with each other in a complex manner, in order to fulfill their varying tasks. Increase in complexity inevitably leads to a propensity to impairment in an environment teeming with menacing microorganisms. This would result in fatal consequences if the organism (i.e., the sum total of all cell agglomerations with their varying functions, control loops, and feedback) had not found ways and means in the course of evolution to effectively combat threats. One of the fascinating examples, and quite simply *the prime example,* is known to everyone, namely the immune system, which will be discussed later. In this context, the flexibility of the systems of control, correction, defense, and/or self-preservation of the organism must be at least as extensive as the wide band of possible attacks (e.g., bacteria and viruses). In single individuals or an entire species, life-endangering situations can arise, with which the organism will be able to cope only after a long period of delay, or not at all. A particularly striking example is AIDS (acquired immune deficiency syndrome), an immune deficiency acquired through viruses, where the defense system itself seems to be the target for attack.

Apart from the illness-causing microorganisms previously considered, there is a multitude of "disturbances," which require difficult tasks of the organism. A continuously unhealthy lifestyle alone can lead to illness. It is well-known and undeniable that poor nutrition (imbalanced; too much sugar; too much fat with high-saturated fatty acids; too few vitamins, minerals, and trace elements), excess weight, lack of movement, persistent physical and psychological stress (smoking, alcohol consumption, excessive sunbathing, experience of personal loss, persistent, excessive demands on oneself, etc.) produce consequences which can take on dramatic forms. Our organism has an astonishing capacity to carry on balancing *adverse* conditions with remarkable *patience* until a *point of no return* is reached, and it falls ill.

One of the most feared illnesses resulting from these *adverse* conditions is cancer, a malignant cell change in its manifold forms, the onset of which is discussed in this hypothesis.

Cancer today occupies third place among the most frequent causes of death in industrialized countries, preceded by infectious diseases and heart/circulatory diseases. The probability that cancer will in the future become the most frequent cause of death increases in proportion with the decrease of the two top diseases, as a result of recent progress, which fortunately achieves a generally higher life expectancy. This unfortunately will increase the probability of living long enough to experience "one's own" cancer.

What Is Cancer?

A clear definition of cancer depends on whether it is viewed solely as the result of an illness developing over many years or whether it includes the full development history with its known stages, which differ in some aspects from those of a healthy person. In general, the first definition is applied, because established methods of primary therapies speak of fighting cancer by attacking malignant cell changes in a direct way. This is not wrong, but I am of the opinion that the problem is not treated in its entirety if cancer is solely regarded as an illness of the genes, leading to malignant tumors, no longer responding to the control, correction, and repair mechanisms (right up to the programmed dying of cells—apoptosis) found in healthy cells. I feel that however important it may be, this narrow fixation on an event taking place on a molecular level is insufficient. In view of the relative difficulty in establishing a point in time from which the definition cancer applies, cancer diagnosis is deemed to have commenced upon confirmation of an existing *aggressive cell proliferation infiltrating adjoining tissues.*

This establishes the most important characteristic, which distinguishes *benign* cell proliferation from *malignant* cell proliferation. Further known differentiation criteria will here be summarized in abbreviated form only. Cancer cells are *potentially immortal*, unless they die prematurely as a result of their own genetic defects. Healthy cells have a finite cell division limit (approximately fifty to seventy times) and need an external command or growth signal in order to divide. Cancer cells *act autonomously, because they do not need such a growth signal.* Healthy cells react to messenger agents of the adjoining tissue, intended to prevent any further division. Cancer cells ignore these signals too. In an extreme case, this leads to *cancer cells bypassing the useful control mechanism of apoptosis*, which is released both from inside a cell (e.g., irreparable DNA damage) or from outside, for whatever reason. Worse still, cancer cells develop the capability to transmit "death messages" against any advancing cells of the immune system, which lead to their dying. They also transmit signals that facilitate the *growth of blood vessels* into tumor tissue and, thereby, establish the necessary structural preconditions for food supply (e.g., glucose), so leading to further growth.

And ultimately, a malignant tumor possesses the life-threatening characteristic of *transmitting daughter cells*, which then infiltrate other separate life-essential organs and form daughter tumors (metastases).

Cancer may show itself in a variety of forms. Today differentiation can be made between approximately one hundred different types of cancer. A malignant primary tumor can start in the lung or in the liver, in breast tissue or in the prostate, in the stomach, intestine or throat, etc. Apart from the heart and most other muscles, there are not many areas that are bypassed by cancer. Differences are recorded in malignancy or speed of growth. In this regard, malignant melanoma is particularly feared. When and where a tumor develops depends on many factors. It is known with certainty that tobacco and alcohol consumption (especially when combined) and unhealthy nutrition carry a high risk. Smoking is the cause of 90 percent of all lung tumors. Observations have shown an almost logarithmic increase in cancer cases with increasing age. Knowledge on so-called virus-associated cancers has grown over recent years. Links have been established between the Hepatitis B virus and liver cancer, papilloma viruses and cancer of the neck of the womb, certain herpes viruses and Caposi's sarcoma, to mention a few examples. In these cases, viruses can directly access and transform the genetic makeup of cell genes or indirectly promote cancer. This touches a point which plays an important role in the hypothesis on the origin of cancer under discussion. Of course, differing, damaging noxae, which are connected with cancer, could also be introduced; however, a hypothesis must also endeavor to explain why some people develop cancer, whereas others don't, despite their being exposed to an identical environment. At this juncture, I will concentrate on generic-regulating mechanisms, the disruption or disablement of which precedes the formation of tumors, whichever risk factors may have given them their fatal chance.

Brief Summary on the Topic of Cancer

A review of the best-known hypotheses on the origin of cancer reveal that enormous progress has been made during recent years of research into the formation of cancer on a molecular level. This probably originated from the desire to find the cancer gene that could be held responsible for the malignant degeneration of cells. Once found, this would have provided a key to conquering the disease. It proved, however, not to be so simple: *there is no cancer gene that can be switched on and off.* Everything turned out to be much more complicated, even chaotic.

The classical approach concentrates on mutations of cancer-associated genes. There are two opposing types of genes: tumor-suppressor genes and growth-stimulating oncogenes. Whereas the former are capable of controlling the rate of cell division and of inactivating cancer-producing mutations, the latter increase the rate of cell division and enable cancer-producing mutations to remain in a continuously active state. Hundreds of these cancer-associated genes have now been identified, which contributes to the difficulty of mapping out accurately the path in the complex interplay of their functions that ultimately leads to the development of tumors. There may even be no such single path, because the system of biochemical regulatory cycles within the cell becomes completely chaotic. Over recent years, the classical dogma that there is a relatively identifiable antagonism between tumor-suppressor genes and oncogenes has increasingly been put in doubt. These doubts are supported by findings showing that many tumors do not consist of a homogenous accumulation of identical, degenerated cells, but of a multitude of genetically differing cells, which would be quite unexpected of a mutation with subsequent cell divisions. Other findings caused even more confusion because they revealed that certain oncogenes in tumors are *less* active than in the healthy adjoining tissue, and yet with some intestinal cancers, a certain tumor-suppressor gene is not inactivated but *overactive*. This stands in contradiction to the classical dogma, which has been branded a failure by a significant number of cancer researchers. The hope of finding *the cancer gene* has, therefore, gone. It has become apparent that entire chromosomes may be present in changed form, or fragmentary only, or even missing altogether. It could even be possible that each tumor is unique in its genetic chaos. And yet there are common factors with tumor cells, striking characteristics, as described above, which make a mockery of the suggestion of an uncontrolled general disintegration of the structure and the functioning of cells.

> At this point, the comments on *reductionism* and *emergence* illustrated at the beginning are more easily understood. It does indeed make a difference whether a problem is tackled on *reductionist principles,* or whether all interrelations are consistently kept in mind, even going one step further and recognizing a *cause-and-effect relationship*. Reductionism requires analyses on ever lower levels right down to the cellular and molecular level of malignant tumors. Such a method may ignore, however, potentially crucial connections and characteristics of a system on higher levels (e.g., impaired hormonal control mechanisms or immunological interactions).

The distinguishing criteria of this hypothesis on the origin of cancer, explained in the following chapter, have already become clear: a different approach to finding a solution, where *higher biochemical regulatory mechanisms play the central role,* and the events on a molecular level a lesser role. It is, of course, necessary to achieve clarification on lower levels as well as on higher levels. The complex cancer process can in my view not be understood in any other way, just like the phenomenon of "life."

The Hypothesis on the Origin of Cancer

Malignant tumors form through insufficiency of the hormone adrenaline. Adrenaline deficiency occurs as a result of accumulated, long-term stress without sufficient physiological release, leading to exhaustion of the adrenaline-producing (chromaffin) system in an over acid and, therefore, cancer-promoting tissue environment, accompanied by a weakened immune system.

Excessive and long-term stress leads to a continuous overproduction of the hormone adrenaline long before the onset of a malignant tumor, finally leading to the gradual dying off of the function of the chromaffin system, which produces the hormones noradrenaline and dopamine as well as adrenaline.

Obviously, adrenaline deficiency in the metabolism has dramatic consequences. In my opinion, this is the *decisive* starting point for the formation of a first malignant cell and subsequent tumors. The life-sustaining importance of adrenaline in the organism is recognized from its tasks:

(1) The first important task is its contribution to the regulation of sugar metabolism. Here, adrenaline is the antagonist of insulin: whereas insulin usually stores any excess sugar in cells (mainly liver cells), adrenaline ensures that sugar is remobilized when required (for muscle work, brain activity, etc.) and made available to the metabolism from the glycogen stored in cells, subsequently yielding glucose.

If adrenaline production dries up, quantities of sugar will be accumulated over a period of time both in the liver cells and subsequently also in other body cells, with a disruptive effect on cell and body metabolism. Normally, excess stored sugar is simply converted into fat by the metabolism, but this is impossible without adrenaline. Noradrenaline, which can also be formed outside the chromaffin system, has no influence on the sugar metabolism and cannot affect the situation.

(2) In times of stress, adrenaline and noradrenaline fulfill important tasks. Adrenaline is capable of coordinating blood vessels, i.e., dilating the vessels

of defined areas of the body and at the same time constricting other areas (by mobilizing alpha and/or beta receptors, i.e., adrenaline-binding and noradrenaline-binding membrane receptors of the response organs of the autonomic nervous system). If this facility fails as a result of adrenaline deficiency, blood vessels within the entire organism are constricted in a one-sided manner by noradrenaline only, leading to a generalized deficiency of oxygen in the body.

Oxygen deficiency and glycogen overloading in a *locus minoris resistentiae* (*Latin*-location of reduced resistance)—in this case a site with a particularly poor blood supply—can lead to a first cell moving over to another reduced type of metabolism (which it is perfectly capable of doing). This is known as fermentation and takes place in the absence of oxygen. It is characteristic of optically levorotatory lactic acid, one of the end products of this type of fermentation (various types are known), to increase eightfold the division of cells in a given time (rate of mitosis), which process again consumes relatively large quantities of sugar. The first small tumor is formed, which draws its energy solely from the fermentation of sugar, and initially relieves the organism. This has created a seemingly logical sugar processing system, which, however, has the fatal characteristic of leading its own life independently of the organism, apart from its permanent requirement for sugar. The cell, its survival for the time being safeguarded by means of fermentation, distances itself from its original purpose within the organism as a whole and, therefore, prepares the way for its destruction.

(3) Adrenaline plays a decisive role as intermediary in the immune defense of the organism. Without it, the immune system is unable to recognize antigens and to fight them. Normally, bacteria, viruses, foreign bodies, etc., release inflammatory defense reactions after each adrenaline discharge. Adrenaline deficiency evidently changes these defense reactions. Tumors are no longer attacked (although they may in any case not react to the immune response) and are able to grow unhindered and ultimately kill off their host.

The following will explain in more detail the hypothesis (in the text often referred to as "the hypothesis" only) outlined above. In its favor is the fact that nearly all experience and theories on malignoma existing to date do not refute it but actually fit easily into it.

My own measurements, taken over many years, of adrenaline production of carcinoma patients have shown that these patients register indeed an extremely low adrenaline level. Initially, I was surprised to find that this was not also true for sarcomas, leukemia, and malignant diseases of the lymph system. All these patients registered rather higher values. Experience furthermore showed these patients to be sympathicotonic, i.e., they may run up a fever and break out in sweat, which is more or less impossible with carcinoma patients. That I was able to cure patients from this group as well is probably due to the fact that their state of chronic overacidification became normalized, and adrenaline, which is extremely pH-value dependent, became effective again.

The reasons for not taking the obvious steps of testing this hypothesis or parts of it on animals were simply a lack of the necessary means and prerequisites (laboratory, material, etc.). Specialist literature[5] points to such experiments, which were, however, carried out only *after* publication of the first edition of my first book on the origins of cancer. They confirm at least a connection, in showing that cancer growth could be hindered or prevented when test animals to which a carcinogen was administered first, or animals that had already developed tumors, were treated either with psycho drugs, which stimulate *adrenaline* production, or with *adrenaline* injections.

"If one administers [. . .] monoamines, such as adrenaline, dopamine, or the monoamine-derivative imipramine, all survive (fifteen rats were used in this test): in the case of imipramine, all were free of tumors."[5]

> The initial research was into how far psycho drugs were helpful with depression. This led to the recognition that they also protect against cancer. In tests with rats, which had been given cancer-stimulating substance—a carcinogen—one group was regularly given over a period of six months the synthetic psycho-drug imipramine (which is similar to the natural stimulants adrenaline and dopamine); a second group received no further treatment. Result: After half a year, eight out of the ten untreated animals had cancer tumors; not a single animal fell ill out of the fifteen animals to which the drug was administered.
>
> Two further groups received the natural stimulants adrenaline and dopamine, and only in two and four cases respectively did cancer tumors form, which grew, however, more slowly than those in the group of untreated animals. "*Sympathomimetic* drugs (i.e., drugs which are equivalent to the natural, sympathetic stimulants) [. . .] and in general agents acting on the central nervous system (CNS), preventing or correcting neurochemical changes in the brain, also prevent cancer growth."

A connection between adrenaline deficiency and the formation of malignant tumors has to my knowledge not been described to date in relevant literature, solely because a hypofunction of the chromaffin system has never been taken into consideration.

This would mean that the chromaffin system would strangely be the sole endocrine gland that merely manages overproduction of hormones—a viewpoint which I found difficult simply to accept, and which was ultimately the starting point for the hypothesis on the origins of cancer here discussed.

The chromaffin system consists indeed of very many anatomical parts, in particular the medullae of both adrenal glands and the chromaffin ganglia (the term *chromaffin* is derived from the fact that ganglia can be visualized with *chromium* dyes) distributed along the sympathetic nervous system, and partial failure can be caused by local damage alone. However, failure as a result of *exhaustion* is known with many other endocrine glands. Why should it, therefore, be different with such an important system as the chromaffin system, if, for example, it is exposed to extreme long-term overload through permanent stress? Stress, be it physical, mental, or infectious in origin (to be discussed later), leads a healthy organism to a discharge of the hormone adrenaline and thereby to a demand on the chromaffin system. Adrenaline puts the organism into a state of alarm, which needs abreaction (i.e., release of tension). It can be safely assumed that in case of permanent stress and absent abreaction—a behavior which goes against "nature" and unfortunately is not uncommon with our modern way of life—the adrenaline-producing (chromaffin) system sooner or later becomes tired and finally breaks down. This has created a first—according to this hypothesis, decisive—precursor, which can lead to the origin of the first malignant cell. This will need further detailed explanation, but first to the hormone which plays the *central role* in the hypothesis.

The Hormone Adrenaline

Generally speaking, hormones have to fulfill extremely varied and vital tasks within the organism. They are the messenger agents, which, in very small quantities (micrograms), produce at a target organ a strong and lasting control effect. Both hypofunction and hyperfunction from the endocrine (secreting into the blood circulation) glands lead to serious disturbances in the organism. The best known are the sex hormones oestrogen or testosterone, followed by the stress hormones adrenaline and noradrenaline or insulin, which alongside adrenaline is absolutely essential for the sugar metabolism.

> The hormone adrenaline was the first among hormones to be isolated in pure form in 1901; also called epinephrine; belonging to the group of catecholamines; chemically: dioxyphenyl ethanol methylamine; produced in the cells of the medullae of the adrenal glands and the cells of the sympathetic nervous system; promotes transformation of glycogen in body cells into glucose in the blood, thereby increasing the blood sugar level; therefore, antagonist of the hormone insulin; has the further task to stimulate the production of free fatty acids in the fat cells; generally known as stress hormone, because it is capable of putting the organism into a state of alarm within seconds of stress situations arising, by increasing the systolic blood pressure, raising pulse frequency, increasing the cardiac minute output, inhibiting gastro-intestinal activity, dilating bronchial tubes and pupils, and leading to a general increase in performance because of promotion of O_2 (oxygen) consumption—a conditioning resulting from evolution in a fight-or-flight situation then followed by abreaction; if this does not take place, the organism will suffer damage sooner or later (e.g., high blood pressure, heart-rhythm irregularities etc.); is used as therapy for allergic shock, cardiac arrest, and as additive in local anaesthetics.

Closer consideration needs first to be given to the most important functions of the hormone adrenaline in the organism and the consequences in case of deficiency.

Sugar Metabolism

In sugar metabolism, the hormone adrenaline is next to glucagon the most important antagonist to the hormone insulin. Insulin builds excess sugar into the cells in the form of glycogen; whereas, in glycogenolysis, i.e., the breaking down of glycogen in the *presence* of oxygen, this sugar is recovered from the cells through the intervention of adrenaline. (It needs to be mentioned at this point that adrenaline also plays an important role in the breaking down of glycogen in the *absence* of oxygen—e.g., as happens in the musculature of the skeleton. The importance of the dissimilation product of *optically dextrorotatory lactic acid* will be discussed later in more detail.)

Adrenaline deficiency consequently results in the stored glycogen remaining in the cells, as it can no longer be mobilized, although in the beginning certain qualifications have to be made. This will be shown later when hormonal substitute reactions are explained that occur in the presence of adrenaline deficiency. The cells are forced to absorb ever more glycogen, as insulin continues to supply sugar, with advanced, malignant illnesses even free, simple sugars. An overload first on liver cells and subsequently on any other cells is the fatal result: a delicate disruption in the cell metabolism and a decisive factor along the way to the transformation of a healthy cell into a malignant cell.

Oxygen Supply

Contrary to general opinion, the hormone adrenaline can not only constrict vessels, but can also coordinate the width of vessels. For example, in case of shock, it functions initially in such a way that less important areas receive a lesser blood supply by a constriction of vessels, whereas important areas receive stronger blood circulation through simultaneous dilation. The task of adrenaline is, therefore, to ensure that emergency areas in the organism receive sufficient oxygen, whereas the chemically closely related hormone noradrenaline in effect always constricts *all* vessels and, thereby, generally throttles oxygen availability.

> The hormone noradrenaline (also called norepinephrine) also counts as a stress hormone; chemically, it differs from adrenaline only by a methyl group; like adrenaline, it belongs to catecholamines; its effects are, however, weaker in part or opposed to those of adrenaline; it is formed and stored not only in the chromaffin system, but also in the synapses of nerve endings, the brain, the mucous membrane of the small intestine and other organs so that sufficient quantities remain in case of failure; it will increase blood pressure but does not improve the pumping strength of the heart; it lowers the pulse frequency and has hardly any or no effect on the blood sugar level; it also reduces gastro-intestinal activity.

Therefore, adrenaline failure, even when a sufficient supply of noradrenaline is still available, will lead to oxygen deficiency in peripheral areas. Cells, which had to fight an extremely overburdened metabolism because of their glycogen overload, would in addition be subjected to oxygen deficiency and slowly die if there were no other reduced kind of metabolism.

Metabolism in Case of Insufficient Oxygen

Many cells have the noteworthy capability to sidetrack from aerobic to the less efficient anaerobic metabolism in the absence of oxygen: more accurately, to make do with fermentation.

The term "aerobic" refers to the metabolic process of a cell which can only take place if oxygen is present and absorbed (respiration). Anaerobic metabolism does not need oxygen. To understand the capability of a cell to change from aerobic to anaerobic requires looking back at evolutionary history.

A criterion for differentiation of organisms is the cell type: there are cells without a cell nucleus (prokaryotes) and cells with a nucleus (eukaryotes) (*Greek: pro* (before), *eu* (true, good); *karyon* (kernel) core). Prokaryotes consist solely of bacteria and blue-green algae; the cells of all green plants and of all animals are eukaryotes. The behavior of prokaryotes in the *presence* of oxygen varies: whereas some cannot exist if oxygen is present, others are capable of tolerating oxygen but can live without it, and others are totally aerobic. Eukaryotes (with very few exceptions) are, however, dependent upon oxygen. From this fact, it can be assumed that prokaryotes are older than eukaryotes, as the first were able to exist during an era when the oxygen concentration in the atmosphere was subjected to constant change, whereas eukaryotes appeared only in the presence of a relatively constant and high oxygen ratio. There is, however, an "evolutionary relationship"[6] in so far as many aerobic cells are capable of restricting themselves to a fermentation metabolism, i.e., anaerobic metabolism, in case of oxygen deficiency.

During fermentation part of the energy released through glucose dissimilation is invested in the form of energy-rich phosphate bonds (usually adenosine triphosphate (ATP) that constitutes *the universal energy store* in biological systems), whereas the rest is lost as heat. Respiration, which requires oxygen, consists, however, of two cycles: glycolysis, followed by the citrate cycle (also citric acid cycle, or a particular Krebs cycle named after its discoverer). During glycolysis, with its low ATP extraction, no oxygen is consumed initially; the citrate cycle that then follows oxidizes carbon atoms and linked reactions finally lead to the synthesis of further

ATP. The entire respiration system is much more productive than fermentation: use of energy is eighteen times as high. The evolutionary relationship can therefore be found in the fact that reaction cycles linked to oxygen do not replace the anaerobic ones, but join them and optimize energy recovery.[7]

Fermentation of sugar into alcohol upon the addition of yeast is a widely known anaerobic biochemical process. More accurately, it is the formation of ethanol from glucose. There are, however, various types of fermentation with differing starting and end products, whereby the end products of some fermentations are the substrates of others. This will, however, not be dealt with in greater detail in this hypothesis.

Louis Pasteur discovered fermentation in the living cell at an early stage (1860). This was for a long time known as vitalistic dogma (French: *la vie sans l'air*, i.e., life without air), until Hans and Eduard Buchner more or less by accident discovered that alcohol fermentation also takes place outside living cells (1897). In the history of evolution, fermentation is the older form of cell metabolism, as free oxygen was not available in the earlier stages of life.

The flexibility of the metabolism (aerobic/anaerobic) attained through evolution is utilized by a cell, when in an extreme case it finds itself in the following situation (as per the hypothesis under discussion, and briefly summarized):

The breakdown of the chromaffin system resulting from continuous stress leads inevitably to adrenaline deficiency. Lack of adrenaline initially leads to an overloading of the cell with glycogen with simultaneous oxygen deficiency in two ways; on the one hand, the vessel-modulating effect of adrenaline fails, but on the other hand, the vessel-constricting effect of noradrenaline continues. The cell "remembers" its early phylogenetic capability of anaerobic, reduced metabolism and reacts precisely in this way. This has, however, ultimately fatal consequences, because the fermentation of glycogen produces optically levorotatory lactic acid, a toxic product for the organism, which increases the mitotic rate (rate of cell division) in the given time span.[8] This mitosis-stimulating effect is perfectly compatible with the idea of an unhindered cell division in case of malignant cells. It gives the organism a further means to rid itself of its excess glycogen in cells: cell nests need a particularly vast amount of glycogen. In this way, the first fermented cell relatively quickly takes on an autonomous form, with the sole goal to use up glycogen. This looks like an efficient utilization of sugar, in the beginning seemingly life-sustaining for the organism, but it results in a toxic end product and increased readiness for cell division with an anaerobic metabolism.

There are also other cells capable of metabolizing glucose independently of hormones and oxygen without the toxic end product of levorotatory lactic acid.

These are muscle cells (with the exception of the heart muscle, which functions more or less entirely aerobically), and erythrocytes (red blood cells, highly specialized components of blood), which indeed cannot become malignant.

Under high demand, muscle cells may need more oxygen than can be supplied by lung and blood, and yet the muscle does not cease to function, because it restricts itself to anaerobic glycolysis by producing optically dextrorotatory lactic acid, which in turn stimulates adrenaline production and has a favorable influence on the acid-alkali household of the organism, as will be discussed later.

> "The occurrence of lactic acid is possibly a remnant of an earlier bacterial metabolism, which was displaced under aerobic conditions."[7] Aching muscles, common after excessive muscle use, are noticeable proof of the presence of, as yet undissimilated, dextrorotatory lactic acid (and alanine) in the tissue.

Erythrocytes use anaerobic glycolysis as their main and even exclusive energy source; for this reason, and because they also have no nucleus, they are comparable with prokaryotes.

> This energy gained per glucose molecule in the form of two ATP molecules is utilized to maintain cell function for as long as possible. Glycolysis, which starts with phosphorylation, ends with pyruvate, which is ultimately broken down into lactate by means of lactate hydrogenation. The intermediary stations are rather complex, and of no further interest in this context.

The Immune System

An organism disposes over a veritable army of various cells and molecules to protect itself against "foreign matter," the best known of which are bacteria and viruses, two of the four large groups of illness-producing microorganisms or pathogens (the other two groups are pathogenic fungi and parasites). Foreign matter also comprises toxins (wasp stings, allergens, etc.), including donated organs (heart, skin, kidney, etc.). The immune system has the task of dealing with anything foreign (unless expressly suppressed—e.g., with drugs—as in the case of transplants with foreign grafts). This is called immune response. Processes where the immune system fights against the body's own substances, i.e., autoimmune illnesses, such as multiple sclerosis or insulin-dependent diabetes will not be considered in this context.

> Today, differentiation is made between congenital and acquired, i.e., adaptive immunity. Congenital immunity fights various pathogens without having met these previously; whereas with adaptive immunity response, only by way of reaction to an infection are antibodies formed, which attack substances grouped together under the collective term antigens. Granulocytes and macrophages (both white blood cells) are largely involved in congenital immunity; lymphocytes (cells maturing in bone marrow and thymus) are involved in adaptive immunity.

Adrenaline is the agent initiating defense processes in the organism, a fact no longer highlighted in authorized textbooks. In addition to its function as a stress hormone as previously described, it promotes the formation of granulocytes and macrophages to combat infections, leading to a rise in temperature, possibly preceded by shivering fits, and the resulting formation of dextrorotatory lactic acid. This in turn promotes adrenaline production, raises body temperature, and starts an acute-type inflammation.

Everybody has at some time experienced an acute infection. The patient usually suffers from exhaustion, painful limbs, sweating, heart palpitation, rise in temperature. In many cases after a given time, the symptoms recede. The organism recovers gradually, and with luck, the infection is overcome without medication. The immune system has managed to cope with the antigen and in some cases (e.g., measles) "learned" to make short work of the same antigen should it be faced with it again. The patient is very often quite unaware of this: he has become immune.

In principle, there are two forms of immune response: cell-transmitted or cellular immunity and antibody-transmitted or humoral immunity (*Latin: humor* (liquid))

> Cellular immune response: if cells become inflamed due to an infection, they are directly attacked during the first phase of the illness by granulocytes (pyosis), followed by a particular type of lymphocyte, i.e., T lymphocytes (T cells) which mature in the thymus. However, as antibiotics are nowadays administered so early to combat infections, inflammations of the acute type can hardly follow their normal course, resulting in a lack of "training" for the immune system. In short, the products of a healthy immune system, namely shivering fits (dispersing large quantities of dextrorotatory lactic acid and consequently stimulating adrenaline production), fever and calor, rubor, dolor (*Latin:* heat, redness, pain) at the site of an infection, are suppressed with great haste. This is more comfortable for the patient, but dangerous in the long term, as such a procedure will over the years lead to the dulling of reactions to any noxae. It makes sense that the subacute defense phase, i.e., the lymphocytic form of immunological response, can only follow after the process of the acute phase of an inflammation has taken place.
>
> Humoral immune response: B lymphocytes (B cells—from bone marrow) discover antigens by means of antibodies on their surface and are then activated.
>
> The exact procedure of every type of immune response is very complicated, as the effective methods of T cells and B cells are closely interlinked. It is intended to show this in brief and schematic form. Macrophages, i.e., cells of the first defense phase of the acute type passing through the body, find an antigen (e.g., foreign protein molecule), ingest it, and break it up into antigenic fragments (peptides) which are bound to molecules of the major histocompatibility complex (MHC) and presented on the cell surface. The T lymphocytes recognize peptide-MHC combinations and are activated to commence division, emit messenger agents (i.e., lymphokines), which in turn mobilize other elements of the immune system, in particular B lymphocytes. These carry receptor molecules enabling them not to acknowledge immediately antigens bound to MHC molecules. Once B lymphocytes are activated, they also divide and consequently produce antibodies capable of attaching themselves to and, thereby, neutralizing the corresponding antigen, and accelerating the

work of the macrophages. Some of the T and B lymphocytes turn into memory cells, which can immediately begin their protective function under renewed contact with the same antigen.[9]

Reaction to inflammations of the acute type comes from the cellular immune response, which in my opinion is capable of coping by itself with degenerated cells. (It is assumed that when the degeneration of cells has reached a certain stage, this will be recognized by the immune system as *foreign* and, therefore, open to attack.) This brings me back to the cancer hypothesis.

> Some theories contend that lymphocytes are continuously on patrol to locate degenerated cells for early destruction. These theories make reference to the relative rise in cancer, e.g., cancers of lung, skin, colon, prostate, breast, or uterus after immune suppression by means of drugs (e.g., after transplants).
>
> Tests on animals have shown that at least some tumors release a specific immune reaction. It is also known that with virus-associated tumors, immune system monitoring can be of use. The present view is, however, that most tumors produce no special antigen proteins and do not build up any stimulating molecules on their surface, which is the prerequisite for setting off an immune response. This conclusion was based on the observation that individuals with a deficiency in T cells do not develop any more tumors than do others.[10]
>
> Other research[11] indicated that protection against attacks on the immune system consists of a halo of hyaluronan. This protection simultaneously increases the adherence of tumors, leading to a greater infiltration of tumors into the tissue and in particular into blood vessels, thereby increasing the migration rate of these invading cells, i.e., the chances for metastases. The possibility for changing these conditions is afforded by parenteral (injected into the tissue) administration of hyaluronidase, with the result that the hyaluronan is broken down.
>
> Fairly, radical cancer immunity therapies also exist, such as the reimplantation of T cells, grown outside the organism, after first conditioning the patient with cyclophosphamide and fludarabine. This first-stage chemotherapy allows the reimplanted, patient-owned T cells to spread in a way that was previously not thought possible, and to attack tumor cells.[12]
>
> In summary, it must be said, however, that the present-day possibilities of immune therapies are relatively modest. In particular, they are not capable of destroying large tumors. Immune therapies are, therefore, largely used to remove tumor remnants after preceding primary therapies. Scientific findings are, however, still in the initial stages.

At this point, the logic of the argument must be kept in mind: adrenaline deficiency as a result of exhaustion of the chromaffin system leads to a change in the cell metabolism (aerobic → anaerobic), *simultaneously* reducing immunological readiness, well before the first malignant cell is formed. Once formed, however, the situation becomes over time so precarious that when neither cellular nor humoral immunity are capable of making an impact, an acute defense will have to be set in motion "from outside." Any doctor who has tried this knows that this is as good as impossible with cancer patients.

Even if it were possible to normalize all defense processes, a tumor would, in my opinion, only be attacked if it had been damaged beforehand so that it can at least function as an antigen by means of the products of its breakup circulating in the blood. Tumor destruction can at present by and large be achieved by means of two methods only: radiation or medication of cytostatically acting substances. However, both methods reduce the defense mechanism immediately after commencement, which makes an immunological destruction of the antigenic products of the breakup very difficult.

The ideal solution would, therefore, be a form of treatment that brings about the destruction of the tumor and simultaneously boosts the defenses. In accordance with the hypothesis under discussion, tumor destruction by means of "starving" the malignant cells should achieve the goal, provided it were possible either to remobilize the adrenaline production of the ailing organism (thereby, mobilizing glycogen out of the cell) or else to stop insulin production (and, thereby, the infusion of glycogen into the cell).

Up to now, no tests have been undertaken to promote adrenaline production in cancer patients; results on the influence of insulin on animal tumors are, however, already available, which would appear to provide positive confirmation of this hypothesis.[13] This will be referred to again in the next chapter.

Insulin Effect

As mentioned before, the hormone insulin is an important antagonist of adrenaline (and glucagon).

> The hormone insulin contributes to the regulation of the carbohydrate metabolism; its antagonists are the hormones adrenaline and glucagon; it is a protein consisting of two chains, produced by the pancreas, lowers the blood glucose level, and plays the decisive role in the treatment of diabetes; initially, proinsulin is produced in the β cells of the islets of Langerhans; this preliminary stage has a third chain that ensures the correct formation of insulin; the level of C peptide, thus, secreted into the blood gives an indication of the activity of the pancreas; normal insulin production amounts to approximately two grams per day; half the insulin is used up in the liver, where some of the glucose is stored; there the most important antagonist to insulin is glucagon, which is produced in the α-cells of the islets of Langerhans in the pancreas, and which ensures the breaking down of glycogen in the liver; worth mentioning is the fact that cortisone is antagonistic to insulin, but analogous to adrenaline, though considerably slower acting.

Adrenaline deficiency causes a relative predominance of the insulin effect, i.e., a kind of hyperinsulinism with all its negative consequences.

It is interesting at this point to consider oncogenes, since the thought arises that the transformation of certain genes in normal cells to oncogenes may be a result of the relative increase of the insulin effect.

Inside healthy body cells are genes that serve to produce enzymes (enzymes are functional proteins that accelerate biochemical reactions in cell metabolism). Only when a "wrong" amino acid is incorporated is the sudden development of a malignant degeneration of the gene and, therefore, the cell set in motion (amino acids are the building blocks of proteins; these are formed from twenty different, natural amino acids). All so-called carcinogens will initially be considered by the hypothesis as the trigger for this transformation. Considering that insulin promotes the process whereby amino acids are built into cells and also their phosphorylation, since it increases the permeability of cell membranes[13][14] coupled with a simultaneous increase in enzyme production inside the cell, this is perfectly compatible with the process of degeneration. "The transition to carcinogenesis is presumed to result from the increased formation of proteins, coded by oncogenes, [. . .] the gene product probably being an enzyme sited at the internal plasma membrane, the function of which is as yet unknown."[15] It is, however, known that just such an enzyme sited at the inner cell membrane transmits the insulin effect from the cell membrane into the inside of the cell, as insulin itself does not penetrate into cells.[14]

The increased incorporation of amino acids and, therefore, the increased protein synthesis inside the cell with the resulting increased enzyme synthesis are, in the opinion established from oncogene research, a cause for the transformation into malignancy. These very characteristics are specific to an excessive insulin effect and point to (relative) adrenaline deficiency.

In other words, the predominance of insulin in the metabolism is the catalyst that allows the mutation to oncogenes of genes that codify the cell signal-transmitting systems, possibly leading to illnesses, and in particular cancer. It is, furthermore, known that insulin causes damage to lysosomes (organelles that are capable of breaking down and reusing damaged cell parts), thereby, hindering or disrupting an important cell repair process.

This is the point where the existing hypotheses on the origins of cancer converge. A multitude of damaging noxae can of course lead to the formation of malignant cells. These can, however, only become active after a lengthy period of functioning as stressors, leading to failure of the defense mechanism of the organism. Normal, healthy defense equates with *adrenaline discharge*.

Literature provides reports on the influence of insulin on tumors. Some findings, gained partly from animal tests, seem to confirm the hypothesis here presented; others seem to contradict it. I will endeavor to resolve this contradiction.

My starting point is this: less insulin means slower tumor growth (relatively, in the case of adrenaline deficiency); more insulin equals faster tumor growth. This is initially confirmed as follows:

"Various transplantable mouse tumors grow more slowly on diabetic mice than on nondiabetic or insulin-treated animals."

"Insulin withdrawal terminates all growth in a human mamma-carcinoma cell, temporarily halting the growth of the small surviving fraction."

There are, however, also seemingly contradictory statements such as "the transplantable R3230 mamma-adeno carcinoma of a rat is inhibited by insulin and then grows faster on diabetic animals."

"Some clinical research shows a relationship between diabetes and endometrial carcinoma; other studies contradict the hypothesis that diabetes is a risk factor for breast cancer."[16]

The last two citations seem to contradict the summary of the first two. This is, however, no longer the case if the possibility is examined that onset of diabetes was not caused by *insulin deficiency* but by *adrenaline deficiency*, which in my opinion applies to most cases of age-related diabetes. I am in no doubt that too much insulin means cancer growth; no insulin means standstill of growth. However, an excess of insulin can only be formed under the right conditions; for *some reason*, the blood sugar level does not fall after discharge of normal quantities of insulin, and insulin will be discharged for as long as the blood sugar level remains high. In accordance with the present hypothesis, the *reason* for the impeded breaking down of the blood sugar is found in the *glycogen overload of many cells as a result of insufficient glycogenolytic hormones, in particular adrenaline*. Thus, the illness, which lays the foundation for the formation of the first malignant cell, is nothing more than decompensated adrenaline-deficiency diabetes.

Objections will of course be raised that not all cancer patients suffer from diabetes.

For as long as replacement hormones are present, there will be no diabetes, and when the hormone production has finally shut down, the formed tumor itself will ultimately ensure that sufficient glucose is consumed right up to cachexia. In the meantime, and this is the decisive point, a diabetic metabolism situation can arise simply as a result of glycogen overload of the cells with insulin-stimulating blood sugar buildup.

Publications[17] point out that many cancer patients show a diabetic metabolism situation or have already shown this years before occurrence of the tumor. That tumors need large quantities of glucose is no longer in doubt. This forms part of standard knowledge on the behavior of new malignant formations.

Substitute Reactions in Case of Adrenaline Deficiency

The organism has at its disposal an astonishing flexibility and elasticity so that lack of adrenaline does not immediately lead to a breakdown of the entire cell metabolism. Well before the first malignant cell is formed, substitute reactions take over, the compensatory effect of which can continue for years. What type of substitute reactions can be expected? Further, which side effect can also appear if these substitute reactions are unable to take over the functions of adrenaline in their entirety, as it must be assumed that as a general rule each "building block" of an organism has its basic right to exist, and redundancy is strictly speaking impossible? (By way of illustration: the main reason for our having two eyes and two ears respectively is not to provide us with a spare in case of loss of one of these two organs, but primarily because of the advantages to spatial perception.)

It is relevant to note the *multipurpose principle* of living things, which allows a biological process simultaneously to serve several purposes in an extremely energy-saving manner. One has only to think of the broad spectrum of adrenaline functions, or the discharge, after appropriate stimulation, of sex hormones with their clearly defined purpose, serving at the same time to boost immune defenses and aid stress release.[18] (Mathematically expressed, a 1:n relation and not an n:1 relation, i.e., one for several purposes and not several for the same purpose.) There is a coexistence (symbiosis) among many living things that are specially adapted for mutual benefit: e.g., bacteria living in the intestinal flora, without which man would not be able to live. The multipurpose principle can also be observed between animals and plants to their mutual advantage.

If the idea of substitute reactions in case of adrenaline deficiency were correct, then empirical corresponding proof from cancer patients should be available.

And indeed there is such proof. Every cancer illness follows its own course, i.e., it is accompanied by various substitute reactions, depending on which substitute hormones respond to the patient's adrenaline deficiency.

Thyroid Hormones

The first problem to show up will be the problem of glucose metabolism. If adrenaline fails, insulin loses its natural antagonist. Insulin continues, however, to be formed in sufficient quantity and ensures continuous input of glycogen into the cells, which it would be impossible to remobilize, were it not for thyroid hormones that are capable of taking over this task as well. It must, therefore, be assumed that an organism, which no longer produces adrenaline, will now need to discharge more thyroid hormones to compensate for the lacking adrenaline. Indeed, many cancer patients have a history of an overactive thyroid. However, at the same time, thyroid hormones attack basic life processes. They cause morphological changes at the mitochondria and force the cells to perform uneconomic tasks through higher energy turnover, RNA (ribonucleic acid) synthesis, and similar.[19]

Thus, the overproduction of compensatory thyroid hormones will promote as its side effect the formation of cell changes and so lay the foundation for a possible subsequent, malignant growth.

Of course, in order to stimulate the thyroid to greater productivity in case of adrenaline deficiency, more of the thyrotropic hormone (a hormone stimulating thyroid function) needs to be released from the anterior lobe of the pituitary gland, for which there must be a sufficient supply of iodine. At some point, this compensatory hyperproduction will exhaust itself, and instead of thyrotropic hormone, the trophic hormone LATS (long-acting thyroid stimulator, serum ā-globulin) will be formed. This too might offer an explanation why under electrophoresis the ā-globulin fraction for so many cancer patients is often "inexplicably" raised: could it be an endeavor by the organism to stimulate the exhausted thyroid and the equally exhausted anterior lobe of the pituitary gland?

Adrenal Cortical Hormones

The adrenal *cortical* hormones (glucocorticoids), belonging to the group of steroid hormones, provide a further means of mobilizing glycogen from the cells. It must be assumed that production of these hormones increases from the fact alone that if the adrenal *medulla* (which ensures formation of adrenaline via the chromaffin system) ceases to function, it will most certainly be stimulated by the pituitary gland (more precisely by adrenocorticotropic hormone ACTH). Although it is held that ACTH solely stimulates the adrenal *cortex*, it would be strange if the pituitary gland (or the hypothalamus) had absolutely nothing to do with regulating the important function of adrenaline production. For me, there is no doubt that ACTH not only stimulates the adrenal *cortex*, but also the adrenal *medulla*, i.e., the adrenaline-producing (chromaffin) system. If this has, however, completely broken down and is no longer responding, it can only lead to an overproduction of adrenal *cortex* hormones (glucocorticoids). This endeavor by the organism makes sense not only because glucocorticoids act glycogenolytically, but also because adrenaline, if it were produced, would remain stable only in the presence of cortisol, a glucocorticoid.[14]

An overproduction of glucocorticoids has, however, various side effects: it can lead to hypertonia, truncal obesity, osteoporosis, and diabetic metabolism. These changes can indeed be found in the anamnesis (history of illness, *pre*history of illness) of many cancer patients. As previously mentioned, many carcinoma patients show a marked diabetic metabolism, which could be an indication of increased production of adrenal *cortex* hormones, but could of course also be derived from adrenaline deficiency alone. This is explained by the fact that with normal insulin production, there would very soon be no space available in cells for the continuous input of glucose so that sugar would have to remain in the blood for longer than normal, leading to a disrupted glucose tolerance. It is necessary to reiterate that I am of the opinion that all age-related diabetes is adrenaline-deficiency diabetes. An age-related decrease in adrenaline production has been acknowledged for quite sometime.

Furthermore, there is documentation[20] reporting increased glucocorticoid particles on the surface of malignant cells in cachectic cancer patients.

Although glucocorticoids are capable of mobilizing glycogen from cells, thereby, substituting some part of the adrenaline function, they nevertheless simultaneously lead to a lowering of cellular immunity, atrophy of the thymus and other lymphatic organs, and finally to a reduction in lymphocytes and eosinophiles (granulocytary leukocytes from the bone marrow, the granula of which contain proteins that stain a brilliant orange with the dye eosin) in the peripheral bloodstream.[19,20] All these effects create, however, a situation, which promotes the formation of malignant cells.

Growth Hormone STH

A third means of substituting adrenaline could come from the overproduction of the growth hormone STH (somatotropic hormone). This hormone has a pronounced insulin antagonism,[14] and its glycogenolytic effect is proven. Unfortunately, the discharge of this hormone also leads to excessive mitosis stimulation, i.e., increased cell division.

Glucagon

Finally, there is a fourth hormone available to the organism, glucagon, which can set glycogenolysis in motion, and has previously been mentioned as an antagonist of insulin. However, glucagon discharge stimulates insulin production so vigorously that glycogen is built back into the cells in larger quantities than before.[14][19] As the hypothesis considers a glycogen overload in the cells to be the cause of malignant growth, its effect would be extremely counterproductive and damaging.

Summary of Substitute Reactions

All substitute hormones that are capable of compensating the glycogenolytic effect of adrenaline have the additional effect—particularly in overproduction—of enabling the formation of a first malignant cell, thereby, advancing a cancer disease. The condition during the phase of precancerosis, i.e., during the period prior to the formation of the first tumor cell, is, therefore, that adrenaline deficiency has led to excessive production of glycogenolytic substitute hormones. It is irrelevant in which order these substitute reactions have taken place: perhaps initially too many thyroid hormones until the thyroid becomes exhausted, then too many corticosteroids until atrophy of the adrenal cortex sets in, then too much glucagon until this too can no longer be produced, and finally too much STH leading to atrophy of the anterior pituitary lobe.

Because of an excess of thyroid hormones and STH, cell division has been promoted; because of too many glucocorticoids, the adrenal cortex / thymus (lymphocytic organs) defense has ceased to function. The granulocytic defense, which depends on a healthy discharge of adrenaline, is similarly spent; oxygen supply to tissues is reduced because of a relative surplus of noradrenaline and consequent capillary restriction; the cells are literally at rupture point with glycogen/glucose; the cell membranes have become permeable because of excess insulin. Now that the organism is more or less defenseless, viruses and other damaging noxae can penetrate damaged cells nearly unhindered, where they rupture the lysosomes or, in the case of viruses, mycoplasms or even bacteria, etc., and transfer their single-cell code into the cells. This alone would be enough to explain why a cell suddenly changes its metabolism and degenerates into a cancer cell which functions autonomously, a behavior that is usually found only in single-celled organisms.

A further factor is that glucocorticoids, STH, glucagon, and also noradrenaline promote lipolysis (fat utilization toward production of energy), thereby promoting the formation of atheromatosis, which in turn leads to a progressive deterioration of blood circulation, i.e., oxygen deficiency in tissues.

Most probably, the same picture emerges with common age-related diabetes (see chapter on insulin). Adrenaline deficiency makes further storage of glycogen in the cells impossible: the resulting increase in blood sugar leads to overproduction of insulin, as known from many cases of age-related diabetes (so-called insulin resistance). Age-related diabetes is, thus, a state of adrenaline deficiency, where, however, sufficient substitute hormones are still being produced.

Paraneoplastic Hormone Changes

Paraneoplastic hormone changes are well-known in medicine. I am convinced that these hormone changes strongly substantiate the cancer-formation hypothesis here presented.

> Paraneoplastic symptoms are hormone changes, which start in humoral manner either from a tumor or one of its metastases, or from one of the body's wrongly coded hormone glands. Such hormones, or polypeptides acting as hormones, cause metabolic or degenerative changes in related organs. Examples are thromboses with pancreatic carcinoma, and hypercalcemia with urogenital carcinoma.

It is assumed that the above-mentioned hormones are often formed in an amine-precursor uptake and decarboxylation organ (APUD), which consists of cells of neuroectodermal origin. These are distributed over the entire body and have an unlimited capacity to absorb and decarboxylate amines or their precursors. If these hormones are considered in greater depth, it very quickly becomes clear that these are side or consequential effects of adrenaline deficiency leading to the onset of a malignant illness.

- **ACTH:** Overproduction of the adrenocorticotropic hormone is to be expected if the pituitary gland endeavors to restimulate the chromaffin system. In contrast to previous opinion and in line with more recent findings, the hypothalamic-hypophyseal portal system stimulates not solely the adrenal cortex system, but also the chromaffin system.
- **Growth Hormone:** Overproduction is to be expected with adrenaline deficiency, as growth hormone acts glycogenolytically, enabling it to substitute in part any adrenaline deficiency.
- **Thyrotropin:** The thyrotropic, i.e., thyroid-stimulating hormone, also acts glycogenolytically and in hyperproduction is capable of counterbalancing adrenaline deficiency.

- **Calcitonin:** An overproduction of thyrotropin has the side effect of forming excess calcitonin, also formed in the thyroid, which lowers the blood calcium level by restricting calcium release from the bones and by increasing calcium discharge in the urine. The preservation of calcium homoestasis of the organism is, thus, disrupted.
- **Follicle-Stimulating Hormone** and
- **Luteinising Hormone:** Overproduction is to be expected with both these hormones as a side effect of overproduction of anterior pituitary hormone.

Also of interest at this point is the ectopic formation of erythropoetin. This is a logical measure by the cancerous organism, as in case of adrenaline-deficiency formation of more erythrocytes offers a very good facility for breaking down glycogen. In addition to muscle cells, erythrocytes (*red* blood cells) are the only cells capable of glycolysis, i.e., breaking down of glycogen without the assistance of oxygen and hormones.

It is a strange fact that in blood samples from leukemia patients the blood sugar level continues to drop for a long time after the sample was taken. Blood sugar values measured two hours after a sample was taken from the patient are considerably lower than the actual value in the bloodstream or the value obtained with immediate measurements. This confirms that the malignant cells of the *white* blood picture have also acquired the capacity to break down glycogen in the absence of adrenaline function. The ectopic formation of hormones, therefore, provides a form of auxiliary assistance in the breaking down of excess glycogen.

Hypoglycemias occurring in patients with large tumor masses also fit into this picture: large tumors, which according to the hypothesis are nothing else but a large sugar-processing plant, no longer take the organism into consideration and consume larger quantities of sugar than the organism can supply to maintain their now autonomous metabolism. This explains the increasing (tumor) cachexia of such patients (emaciation of the organism through malfunctioning of various organ functions). Nearly all of the above-listed ectopically formed hormones have at the same time a lipolytic effect so that if the tumor lacks glycogen for maintaining its metabolism, it ultimately requires free fatty acids to be made available. And finally, many of the above-listed ectopically formed hormones have an anti-insulin effect, which hinders the input of glycogen into cells.

Whereas at the commencement of a cancer illness, i.e., at a time when the tumor mass is still relatively small, cells are overloaded with glycogen, in the end, the tumor uses up all the sugar and on top of that the energy reserves of its host. The situation at the beginning, because of the small capacity of the "sugar-processing plant," is diabetic metabolism that causes the existing sugar to remain in the blood for longer. The cells are engorged with glycogen and can no longer take on more sugar, even if more insulin is discharged. The end effect is an enormous demand for energy that can no longer be satisfied, ultimately resulting in cachexia.

Acid-Alkali Household

As has been demonstrated, adrenaline or the lack of it plays the central role in this hypothesis. As its stability and effect in the organism are only guaranteed at a blood-pH value of 7.4, the relevant aspects of the acid-alkali household of the organism need to be discussed.

> The pH value (Latin: *potentia hydrogenii* [hydrogen concentration]) measures the concentration of acids and alkalis. Measured values are on a scale of between 0 and 14, the neutral point for water being the middle value of 7. The more acid, the lower the pH value; the more alkaline, the higher the pH value. Acids and alkalis have opposing chemical reactions, but brought together, they form neutral salts. A healthy body functions mainly in the alkali range. There are, however, significant deviations: gastric juices, for instance, are strongly acidic, with a pH value of between 1.2 and 3.0; urine can fluctuate between 4.8 and 8.0; muscles at 6.9 lie in a slightly acidic range, because they are nearly continuously active. In this context, the balance between blood-pH value and tissue-pH value will be considered further.

The organism of a healthy person registers a blood-pH value of approximately 7.4 and a slightly more alkaline tissue-pH value of up to 7.7. The body always endeavors to maintain this slight difference by means of complex metabolic processes (buffering, formation of salts, etc.), which ensures that all cells function smoothly in their finely tuned and balanced interaction. The laws of nature state that changes of the pH values of both blood and tissue are in inverse proportion, i.e., if the pH value of the blood becomes more acid, the pH value of the tissue becomes more alkaline and vice versa.[21]

Longer-lasting malfunctions of the acid-alkali balance consequently lead to damage of various cells. If, for example, extreme acid buildup in the intestine leads to protracted overacidification of the blood, the products of excessive acid metabolism that cannot be excreted are stored in the tissue so as to ensure at least a normal blood-pH value. Increasing overacidification of the tissue can sometimes result in restriction of cell respiration[22] and, thereby, a slowing down of the cell-metabolism processes, with accumulation of pathological cell-metabolism products. For example, formation of salts can lead to the formation of stones (gall and kidney stones, gout, etc.). As an increase in relative overacidification of tissue leads to an increase in relative alkalization of the blood (according to the laws of nature mentioned above), the consequences are an increasing malfunctioning of the hormone household (hormones are to a high degree dependent on the presence of a given blood-pH value). This provides a starting situation for a wide variety of illnesses, one of them being cancer.

It would go beyond the framework of this book to deal in greater detail with the complex principles of research into pH values. It is intended only to draw essential conclusions from these brief notes on the acid-alkali household and to argue that nearly all chronic illnesses, including malignant diseases, would be curable if it were possible to reestablish the normal ratio between blood pH and tissue pH. At this point, it becomes particularly clear that a cancer illness has a long prehistory and that several factors play a part at any one time. The acid-alkali household touches on the central point of the hypothesis—adrenaline deficiency—in so far as the stability and efficiency of adrenaline is only given at a blood-pH value of around 7.4. As described in the chapter "Therapy," my first endeavor is to reestablish a healthy acid-alkali balance, whereby optically dextrorotatory lactic acid plays the decisive role.

> The terms "optically dextrorotatory" and "optically levorotatory" refer to optically active substances, which rotate the plane of polarization in a clockwise or anticlockwise direction respectively, when viewed in the direction of travel of the light.

This is demonstrated by nature itself: all kinds of movement usually produce dextrorotatory lactic acid (glycolysis in the muscle), which can be said to physiologically restimulate adrenaline production by "reporting" that glucose is now needed in the muscle. The appearance of dextrorotatory lactic acid in the blood leads to discharge of adrenaline, to glycogenolysis, and (from everyday experience) also to a rise in temperature, dilation of capillaries, increase in heart rate, improvement in oxygen availability, in short to an increase in metabolism promoting cell respiration, and consequently faster elimination of pathological, acidic metabolism products from the tissue. This is common sense but does not fit well in the modern way of life with little physical activity. Exercise, in the open air if possible, helps to maintain health. This takes on a specific importance in the hypothesis on the origins of cancer under discussion.

A side effect frequently observed with cancer patients is obvious, debilitating chronic fatigue, which far exceeds mere tiredness. The *Sahlgrenska Academy in Gothenburg (Sweden)* has published a broad study[23] on cancer-related fatigue. Of interest are the medical recommendations for alleviating apathy, lack of drive, and depressive mood swings brought on by fatigue. A certain degree of physical stress was considered helpful: "Cancer-related fatigue should not as a rule be met with excessive rest. Sports activities and treatment with erythropoetins in cases of diagnosed anemia are the sole measures which indeed relieve the exhaustion. Recommended exercise activities are aerobic training, walking on the treadmill, or nonstrenuous cycling. Depending on the type of illness and on the patient's condition, light power training might be beneficial."[24] As can be seen, there is a striking correlation between adrenalin deficiency, overacidification of the tissue, and fatigue. If muscle work brings relief, then this is linked to stimulation of adrenaline discharge. One could say activity is always a good thing, and this a trivial point. This may be true, but, although for a number of illnesses rest is absolutely essential, here muscle activity and cancer are expressly brought together in a positive relationship. This relationship exists, although it is not (yet) clearly understood. The cancer-formation hypothesis presented herein offers a plausible explanation.

Physical activity is also advisable to counteract the intensification of stress, a further important factor in the hypothesis.

Stress

This chapter brings us a step nearer to the phases of cancer formation. For better understanding of the hypothesis, it is important to clarify some basic definitions. The next decisive point in the cancer-formation hypothesis is stress, a much-discussed phenomenon of modern lifestyle. In the colloquial sense, the term "stress" is usually used to describe a condition where we are faced with unpleasant, taxing demands. To my knowledge, the word is ascribed to Hans Selye,[25] who himself pointed out the inconsistent use of this terminology.

> Many years later, a somewhat sarcastic comment by the publisher of the *British Medical Journal*—namely that in Selye's opinion stress had its own cause—drew my attention to this regrettable error [. . .] I should have differentiated between stress and that which causes stress. I should have spoken of biological "strain," which is caused by biological "stress." However, by then it was too late to change the terminology [. . .] I, therefore, decided to introduce an English neologism, namely the word "stressor." In this way, I was able to retain the terminology of "biological stress" for the reaction, which was how it had been generally used, and use "stressor" for the generating agent.[25]

The designations stress (for exertion, strain, pressure, overload, nervousness, physical alarm) and stressor (for the stress trigger) are today accepted in general use and in research, although varying definitions, theories, or models exist.

> According to *Cannon's* stress theory (1932), stressors lead to a so-called fight or flight syndrome, i.e., the organism is readied for either defensive aggression or for flight through a sudden discharge of the stress hormones adrenaline and noradrenalin. The physiological processes taking place at that time have already been described.

Selye's stress theory (1957) describes the general adaptation syndrome, which is divided into three phases: alarm reaction, resistance phase, and exhaustion phase.

Only some of the existing further models will be mentioned here:

— the cognitive model by *Lazarus* (1974) which contains three stages of stress processing. First, recognition and assessment of the risk of a situation, followed by an evaluation of anticipated somatic harm, psychological losses, and psycho-social cost. Parallel with this, available alternatives for overcoming the situation are considered, such as attack or flight, altering of conditions, negation of the situation. Finally comes a new evaluation of the changed position, which can lead to pathological adaptations;
— the stress model as per *Janke*. This model has in the center a black box, in which stressors are recognized and processed. How this is done depends on certain personality characteristics and can be observed as reaction on a physiological, psychological, and behavioral level. Why stressors are interpreted as irritants depends furthermore on general personality factors (e.g., neuroticism).

In general, it can be said that every situation in life that makes special demands on our adaptive mechanisms, whether physical or psychological, generates stress. There is no such thing as stress-free life, and we need stress to live. This shows that it is an equilibrium phenomenon: excessive stress (hyperstress) is just as damaging as to little stress (hypostress). Furthermore, there is good stress (eustress: G*reek eu* (good, true)) and its counterpart (dis-stress). Everybody is familiar with situations of happy excitement, even euphoria, or paralyzing frustrations, even depression. It is not difficult to see that dis-stress is more likely to cause sickness than eustress, and the likelihood of falling ill increases the longer dis-stress lasts. Temporary dispositions, leading to differing reactions in comparable situations, also play a role in addition to personality characteristics, but this will be discussed later. A factor, which on one occasion can lead to a rising or lowering of the eustress/dis-stress level, can on another occasion have the reverse effect. Striving for success and finally achieving the goal is in many cases very satisfying. The pressure of success, the buildup of unacknowledged, excessive demands on oneself, followed later by a kind of melancholy over its achievement, may leave a damaging overlay on the feel-good factor. The daily jogging routine, initially promoting eustress, can turn into dis-stress, in the same way that transcendental meditation can become torturous boredom, if not properly understood.

It is not intended to delve deeper into this topic; the sole purpose is discussion of stress and its consequences in so far as they are relevant and important for the cancer-formation hypothesis. For this, I will closely follow the theories of Selye, as the development of a cancer illness over many years in my opinion corresponds with the Selye syndrome (general adaptation syndrome), which consists, briefly summarized, of three phases:

The first phase, alarm reaction, is marked by initial incapability to adapt. This leads to shock with a drop in blood pressure, thickening of the blood, and increased capillary permeability. Shock is followed by countershock with adrenaline discharge, shivering fits, rise in blood pressure, and rise in temperature.

The second phase, the resistance phase, is marked by optimum adaptation, formation of immune complexes, adaptation of blood circulation, etc.

The third phase, exhaustion, leads to necrosis in the adrenal cortex, involution of the thymo-lymphatic mechanism, formation of stomach/intestinal ulcers, etc.

The third phase is of particular importance. I am in no doubt that an essential factor of the exhaustion syndrome is the drying up of adrenaline production as a result of exhaustion of the chromaffin system. This is the axis and anchor point of the cancer-formation hypothesis. It can be said with certainty that continuous stress causes atrophy not only of the cortex of the adrenal gland, but in particular of the overstressed medulla, including the chromaffin ganglia.

The cause of stress, i.e., the stressor, can be external (nicotine, asbestos, intense UV light, radioactive radiation, etc.), infectious (retro viruses, etc.) or psychological (major misfortunes). Doubts were cast on the effect of the latter until the beginning of the 1980s when a new branch of science was set up: psycho-neuro immunology, shortly followed by psycho-neuro immuno oncology, which in short established the connection between the centers of the cerebrum (the psychological center) and, for example, the autonomic centers of the organism.

The anamnesis of cancer patients frequently shows experience of great misfortunes or other conditions that placed a burden on the patient over a long period, until a final, unbearable event brings out into the open a cancer that had been developing in that time. Proof from specialist literature: "a significant weakening of cellular immune function was noted in trials with twenty-six persons six weeks after the death of a spouse. Persons with high stress and few symptoms showed the highest, and persons with high stress and pronounced symptoms the lowest NK *(natural killer cells)* activity."[26] Tests on animals point in the same direction: "Riley described a preventative function of stress reduction in mice in relation to the formation of breast cancer in female mice. Mice kept under stress under laboratory conditions showed 80 percent to 100 percent more breast cancers after one year. Only 10 percent of animals from the same breed developed tumors under reduced stress, providing clear proof of a relationship between stress and the plasma-corticosterone level. Destruction of circulating T lymphocytes and thymus involution as a result of increased cortisone production were stated as reasons for reduced immune competence.

In the context of the hypothesis here presented, the question of whether a stressor is of a type that has a long-term or intermittent effect on the organism only plays a subordinate role. In the end, they all lead to exhaustion of the chromaffin system and, therefore, to a decrease of adrenaline production until final failure. Theories that fit into this picture are the virus theory (the so-called slow viruses are in particular regarded as permanent stressors), the theories of chronic irritation (lip cancer in pipe smokers, Schneebergian lung cancer, silicosis, cancer in chimney sweeps and asbestos workers, etc.), the theory of the trigger role of nicotine, and hereditary theory (a weak chromaffin system can be hereditary or acquired in the infant stage through not being fed with mother's milk).

The hypothesis that chronic foci of suppurations contribute to the formation of malignant illnesses is also understandable in that such foci force the organism continuously to take local defense measures until the chromaffin system is exhausted.

> The term "stress" is also found on the molecular level. Recent research provides interesting connections with the above observations. The fairly young science of molecular epidemiology talks of oxidative stress, relating to a molecular process directly connected with unhealthy nutrition, with smoking, with chronic inflammations, and also with asbestos or heavy metals such as iron and copper. It is always a matter of extremely reactive molecules, so-called free radicals, that are capable of laying the foundations for faulty interpretation of cell division by oxidizing DNA bases. This is normally kept in check by the body's own enzymes or antioxidants (vitamins C and E); however, if present in excess, they promote malignant aberrations.

Some notes on the situation of a person who in the middle of an active life is suddenly confronted with the diagnosis of cancer: This is like hearing one's death sentence. After a prolonged period under stress, a person now has to face exponential progression of his stress: now increased by fear for his life, worry about having to undergo a therapy requiring the strength that comes of desperation, therapy with no certainty of success, and a host of other doubts or worries that may release deep depression. In such a situation, where one's existence moves to the very edge, the first requirement should be total avoidance of psychological (and of course physical) stress, but the helplessness of the situation promotes just the opposite. Added to this will be a high degree of further physical stress if the patient decides to undergo primary therapy. Both surgery and radiotherapy, and also chemotherapy, are such radical interventions into the organism that hyperstress resulting from such treatments causes a momentary total paralysis of the defense functions. (Sometimes such measures are, however, successful, and a so-called shock therapy can remobilize the chromaffin system—but there is no guarantee.)

If after all the patient has survived these interventions, his life from now on will be burdened with a new kind of dis-stress: lower self-esteem, completely changed way of life, and worst of all the fear of a relapse, which can happen with all types of cancer. There is a great danger of getting stuck in a vicious circle where the new worries act as stressors and lead to a deterioration of the condition, perceived by the patient as life threatening, which reinforces the worries, etc. (increased stress reactivity). Expressed euphemistically: the "lightness of being" (to paraphrase *Milan Kundera*) is gone once and for all.

In my opinion, it becomes clear at this stage how important it is to understand the formation of cancer and to draw appropriate conclusions. This is normally completely ignored with primary therapies. It is not intended to belittle these, but in the final analysis, any surgical interference is always a palliative measure only (alleviation but not healing of an illness). (It is doubtful whether someone can be declared "free of metastases," when it is known that in order to show up on x-rays or to be felt, a metastasis must have a minimum diameter of 0.5 cm, but at that size already consists of millions of cells.)

These are, however, considerations on stress at a point in time when other stressors have been effective over many years and have led to the grievous illness that is cancer. A therapy on the basis of the presented hypothesis is not simplified by the knowledge of these connections; however, in my opinion, it is more likely to offer success.

Is There a "Typical Cancer Personality"?

Where tumors run in families, it appears likely that hereditary gene defects are the cause. This is for example true for some intestinal cancers (hereditary adenomatous polyposis causes the development of many polyps in the colon, which can turn malignant). Hereditary traits are also possible with breast cancer. This chapter will, however, not deal with such cases but concentrate on character traits.

Ancient Greek teaching distinguished between four personality types. The doctor and philosopher *Hippocrates* (460-377 BC) called these choleric, melancholic, phlegmatic, and sanguine and linked them not only to the cosmic elements of fire, earth, water, and air, but also to corresponding body fluids, namely yellow bile, black bile, phlegm, and blood. Hormones and stressors were then not known, but the view then held that black bile makes people melancholic is worthy of note, as it establishes a psychological-physiological relationship. In medieval times, it was believed that a person with cancer would be rather a depressive and "slower" type, and black bile was also mentioned as a contributory factor to this characteristic.

Today, every experienced cancer therapist will confirm that cancer patients show typical personality traits. The double-sided question, therefore, arises: Is it possible to map out a personality that in all likelihood *will fall ill with cancer in future*, as against a different personality but with similar lifestyle; or can this character comparison be made only between a person who has already developed cancer, as against a randomly chosen healthy person?

Nowadays, two anxiety types are recognized in *healthy* individuals: vagotonic and sympathicotonic (*Latin: tonus* (state of excitement)). The differences in the reaction pattern under stress situations are clear: a vagotonic character shows an overreaction of the parasympathetic nervous system resulting in reduced heart and respiration rates, slackening of muscle tension, and so on (comparable with the submissive posture and playing dead by animals); a sympathicotonic character shows activation of the sympathetic nervous system, with increase in readiness to fight or take flight and increased heart, respiratory, and circulatory activity. One type (*feminine*) reacts to the situation with near unconsciousness and paralysis, while the other type (*masculine*) actively attacks the threat, fully mobilized. (I can foresee protests, but I deliberately chose the differentiation between the sexes, as vagotonic is more closely associated with females and sympathicotonic more appropriate for males.) These differing characteristics can no doubt be explained by evolution, in that they offer clear advantages (some aggressive animals leave a victim alone if it signals either submission or plays dead; with others, a speedy escape or killing before being killed are the best courses of action). This points to a genetic inheritance, added to which are overlying or subliminal cultural and environmental factors. Such behavior patterns alone are in my opinion insufficient to promote cancer; the decisive factor lies in the psychological-physiological processes of stress management during and after the long-lasting effects of stressors on both these character types. Sympathicotonic characters seem to have an advantage, simply because their stress management strategies are more favorable.

As regards "cancer personality," it can best be said that this develops in the course of the illness in a typical way: as long as adrenaline, and subsequently substitute hormones such as thyroid hormones, are produced in sufficient quantity, each patient will be different. If, however, the hormones stimulating the sympathetic nervous system subsequently fail, then the now-typical cancer personality develops: strikingly stoical, nonaggressive, enduring and carrying his/her suffering in an astonishingly disciplined manner and having forgotten how to express true feelings and fears. The person has become vagotonic, even if *he/she had not been so before.* After successful therapy—a therapy that has restarted adrenaline production—complaints are heard that the docile and obedient patient suddenly has become willful and vehemently tries to give himself/herself a new direction in life. These are typical sympathicotonic characteristics (however, patients with sarcoma (tumors of connective tissue origin) or leukemia indicate *no* adrenaline deficiency, and they suffer frequently from fever and breakout in sweat, which fits the model of a sympathicotonic person). If the conversion of a patient from vagotonic to sympathicotonic is successful (even if he never was this type while healthy), then he/she is halfway to being cured.

> Individuals may also be characterized as either introverts or extroverts.[27] Observations have indicated that introverts show stronger physiological reactions to stressors, becoming more tense and self-critical; whereas, extroverts, similar to sympathicotonic characters, tend more to do something to relieve the stress. As regards falling ill with cancer, the same as

above applies to these types also. The decisive factor is stress management of long-acting stressors. If this is not successful or only insufficient, the individual shows to a greater or lesser degree the same characteristics of introversion or vagotony, which are the result of the physiological causes under discussion.

Phases of Cancer Formation

We have now assembled all the pieces that are needed for understanding the formation of cancer as per the hypothesis here presented (exhaustion of the chromaffin system caused by stress over a long period, adrenaline deficiency, immune insufficiency, disturbed antagonism between adrenaline and insulin, damaging side effects from the reaction to substitute hormones, paraneoplastic hormone changes, disturbed acid-alkali household, vagotonic disposition). Malignant illnesses can appear like a bolt from the blue in the shape of a tumor, causing the patient to ask why me?; patients believe themselves always to have been healthy and cannot think of any cause for this terrible illness with which they are now faced. (My somewhat-baffling reply to this is "You were never ill, because you have never been healthy.") This "having been healthy" is a typical statement of most patients and, if questioned about their health record, usually they draw a blank. My experience has shown that cancer patients have indeed rarely been really ill, have very rarely experienced serious accidents or undergone surgery. However, further questioning shows repeatedly that approximately fifteen to twenty years before the tumor showed itself, the patient's life had been affected by long-term influences, such as cancer-promoting noxae (nicotine, asbestos, harmful gases, strong UV light, retroviruses, wrong nutrition, etc.) or have been psychologically affected through extreme circumstances. Thus, in most cases, the tumor required such a long time to form. Applying the hypothesis, this means that after exhaustion of adrenaline, all possible substitute reactions were used up by the organism in order to facilitate its continued survival. Only after the irretrievable breakdown of the last of these life-maintaining functions of which the organism is capable as a result of its extremely high flexibility to organize its processes does the tumor get its chance to grow more or less unhindered.

With particular regard to the changes over the years in the immune situation in individuals who develop cancer, various stages occur: the first stage, called *normergy*, is the proper, nonallergic preparedness of the organism to react to an irritation (infection, initial allergen contact, etc.) during which a functioning defense mechanism still responds to an adrenaline discharge (acute-type response), with fever, sweating, granulocytisis, removal of harmful allergens through macrophages, formation of leukocyte interferon and increased metabolism with improved canalization (kidneys, liver, skin) for elimination of accumulated waste products. This is followed by the *allergy* stage: inappropriate reactions resulting from the change from sympathicotonic to vagotonic. In an acute-immune-phase mast cells, lymphocytes and plasma cells now come on the scene instead of granulocytes and macrophages; serotonin is formed as a substitute hormone for adrenaline as the basophil cells and thrombocytes decline. Subfebrile temperatures are still a possibility, but by and large, this reaction is no longer fully sufficient; the organism may also no longer be capable of coping with a harmful agent so that contact with a new agent may often prove fatal. The next stage over a period of further years on the path to cancer shows itself as advanced allergic reaction, called *hypergy*, which can express itself in chronic allergic illnesses (certain types of asthma-related bronchial-cardio spasms, chronic skin allergies, allergic oedema). It is an old adage in the medical profession that someone with an allergy will not have cancer, i.e., for as long as a person is capable of producing allergic reactions, he does not yet have cancer, because a "wrong" defense is still better than none. With the passing of time comes the complete failure by the immune system to respond (*anergy*), with relatively rapid tumor growth and a multitude of symptoms.

An objection may be raised at this point that babies, children, and teenagers can have cancer, although they have not experienced sufficiently long, preceding periods of permanent stress. They also do not easily fit the pattern of the various stages of the formation of cancer. In such cases, the development of the adrenal system needs to be taken into consideration. The chromaffin system is part of the adrenal gland system, for the healthy development of which the first few months in the life of a baby are decisive. Babies of mothers under permanent stress already suffer dis-stress while in the womb, as recent research has shown. Consequently, children of mothers who are unhappy during pregnancy may be more prone to cancer than those of happy mothers. However, infant nutrition plays a more important role: optically dextrorotatory lactic acid in mother's milk enables breast-fed infants to develop a healthy adrenal gland system, which in newborns is not yet fully developed and fully functioning. Until that process is completed, all babies (human or animal) still have a functioning thymus gland, which becomes atrophic after full development of the adrenal gland system at approximately three to eight months. However, in an emergency, the thymus gland can be reactivated. This is the reason why thymus extracts are administered for malignant illnesses. Children who are fed with baby milk products—particularly before they are fully mobile—never have a healthy adrenal gland system and consequently no efficient chromaffin system, simply because the vital dextrorotatory lactic acid is lacking. This leads to adrenaline deficiency, which touches on the core of this cancer-formation hypothesis.

In animal tests on newly born piglets (*G. Scylvay*), a litter was divided into two groups: one group was reared on sow's milk, the other with artificial products. On dissection, the adrenal gland systems of both groups were examined: all artificially reared piglets clearly showed poorly developed adrenal gland systems in contrast to those reared on sow's milk.

The model of the phases of cancer formation cannot be applied to sarcoma or leukemia patients, because they produce sufficient adrenaline, which, however, is not able to be effective because of the nonphysiological blood-pH value.

The Therapy

The starting point of a successful therapy is immediately apparent if the causes for formation of cancer are kept in mind as there are in essence: lack of adrenaline due to the effects of physical, emotional or infection-induced stressors over a long period of time, and overacidification of tissues resulting from poor nutrition and/or an unhealthy way of life (smoking, lack of movement, and others). It is, of course, not possible to develop universal guidelines, as suitable treatment forms depend on many circumstances, such as type of cancer, stage of disease, constitution of the patient, etc., as is well-known to every cancer therapist. In the beginning, I explained that the hypothesis and the therapy differ from classical viewpoints and primary therapies. Here I want to discuss the differences only. Although surgery, chemotherapy, or radiation will not be discussed, this does not mean that they are dismissed from the outset, or categorically excluded, as a prudent (additional) course of action.

The development history of a tumor illness is of course the central consideration. All types of dis-stress (physical, psychological, infectious) must be avoided as far as possible. Of course, this includes smoking, drinking of alcohol, and similar. If adrenaline deficiency is the decisive factor, it follows automatically that a diet must be adhered to which does not burden the chromaffin system.

The Diet

At the top of the list of every internal cancer therapy

- is thorough detoxification of the intestines, which requires the supply of healthy intestinal bacteria.

Rules for the recommended diet are

- free from those carbohydrates that could be built into the cells. Of course, not every type of sugar is prohibited: fructose, invertose, sorbitole, and lactose are immediately metabolized, if not taken in excess quantities; the same is true for pure honey, although it contains several "prohibited" sugars (glucose, dextrose, saccharose); the constituents of honey are, however, optically dextrorotatory and are, therefore, only converted into glycogen if taken in relatively large quantities; honey contains also propolis (a very health-sustaining constituent) and numerous vitamins and trace elements that can have a favorable effect on cancer illnesses;

- as little as possible of (animal) fats with a high proportion of saturated fatty acids; instead, (vegetable) fats with monounsaturated fatty acids (e.g., olive oil, soy oil, wheat germ oil) and fats with polyunsaturated fatty acids that can influence cholesterol metabolism—all in moderation;
- rich in vitamins, minerals, trace elements, and optically dextrorotatory lactic acid;
- plenty of fluid to eliminate toxins: fruit juices are particularly suitable due to their vitamin content and buffer substances. To use mineral water for this task is a common mistake, because it is incapable of flushing out the salts formed in the tissues of a sick person, as osmotically it is highly saturated and cannot, therefore, absorb and discharge salts from the tissue.

A brief reminder of physics: osmotic pressure between two liquids separated by a semipermeable membrane, leading to diffusion through the membrane, i.e., balance of concentration, is restricted if they are of similar concentration (e.g., salt content).

Ordinary bottled drinking water is most suitable and also cheaper. Mineral water should, however, not be completely eliminated, because, as its name implies, it supplies a greater or lesser number of minerals and trace elements (as per the analysis on the label), but it should not form part of the recommended minimum liquid consumption of two litres per day;

- little meat, particularly red meat, so as not to intensify acidification of the tissues; substitution with fish is recommended;
- whole-grain products, which assist intestinal detoxification due to their high content of fiber and B-group vitamins;
- fruit and vegetables—organically grown, if possible—should of course form a large part of the nutrition, all eaten raw wherever possible.

If sufficient movement, in the open air if possible, no nicotine, moderate intake of alcohol, and effective stress management strategies are added to this list, it becomes clear that these recommendations are not very specific and could apply all the time, not only in times of illness with cancer. This is true, but how many people adhere to them? (Prevention of cancer will be the topic of discussion in the next chapter.)

Thorough intestinal detoxification and adherence to the recommended diet initially lead to a fairly rapid loss of weight. This can quickly lead to psychological problems and loss of confidence in the doctor treating the patient, because cancer patients in principle link loss of weight with progression of the illness toward death. In general, a good therapy must fulfill three expectations: the tumor must be reduced, and the marker count (especially metabolism products produced by tumor cells) must decrease; patients do not want to suffer undue pain, nor do they want to lose weight.

This loss of weight has, however, no connection whatsoever with the progression of the illness. It is initially only loss of salt and water from tissues, which is made up after a few months of the therapy through the buildup of new muscle mass. There is no need for this cancer-hostile diet to be low in calories.

Extensive laboratory tests will show which further measures need to be taken. For example, evaluation of electrophoresis: if the albumin level is low, it must be supplemented (infusion of human albumin). If the level of ā-globulin is high, it must also be replaced (e.g., injection of slow-release beriglobin), as an increased reading points to immune-insufficient paraglobulins.

Persons with tumor illnesses nearly always suffer from iron-deficiency anemia, for which a therapy with iron preparations is advisable in most cases. In the same way as iron, other minerals, such as calcium, potassium, and magnesium, must be supplemented if a deficiency has been established. Cell metabolism depends to a large extent on the exchange of these minerals. In an overacid organism, however, these are substantially used up in the formation of salts and are, therefore, lacking. The same applies if there is a deficiency of zinc, copper, or selenium, which need to be supplemented.

It must, however, be pointed out that the measured values of the blood serum do not always show the true picture. It is possible that a deficiency exists in tissues, which does not (or not yet) show up in the blood serum (for instance normocalcaemic tetany, a syndrome of heightened excitability of motor nerves through deficiency of nonbound Ca^{2+} ions). It is, therefore, absolutely essential also to rely on clinical symptoms.

Attention must of course be paid to the marker values, because nearly all patients base their well-being or otherwise on these metabolism products specifically produced by tumor cells. *If the marker values drop, the patient is happy; if they increase, his world collapses*, because he was told that an increase in the values indicates tumor growth, whereas a drop indicates remission. What the patient was not told, however, is that markers can rise to an extremely high level when the tumor disintegrates! When this occurs during therapy, both the patient and the doctor treating him are horrified and advise immediate resort to "conventional" surgical measures.

An extreme and completely normal increase in marker values when a tumor disintegrates occurs with this therapy in approximately 60 percent of cases, during the fourth month of treatment. It is caused by an inflammatory attack against the tumor cells, which will show up in laboratory results: erithrocyte levels rise; the leukocyte count increases; LDH, alkaline phosphatases, and ā-GT levels rise; the red blood count can deteriorate, also the results of the liver test.

More or less without exception, these symptoms are indicative of an "enlargement" of tumors and recede of their own accord after approximately two months. During this period, the patient will experience no more than the *calor-rubor-dolor syndrome* of an acute inflammation. It is sometimes also necessary to promote discharge of the resulting disintegration products by means of liver infusions.

Acid-Alkali Ratio

This section is devoted to the acid-alkali ratio between tissue and blood. A cancer patient always suffers from overacidification of the tissues, i.e., a clear reversal, to varying degrees, of the pH-value ratio of tissue and blood, compared with a healthy person. In order to deprive the tumor of a favorable environment, the tissue-pH value must be changed from acid to alkaline. This is easier said than done because all alkaline-forming nutrition loses its intended effect soon after entering the bloodstream, as it is used up in the blood for buffering, i.e., before it can reach the tissue. The organism always endeavors via appropriate regulating mechanisms to maintain the blood-pH value at around 7.4, which is absolutely essential for the stability of hormones, in particular adrenaline, as previously demonstrated. A brief recapitulation of the law of reversed proportionality of pH value changes in tissue and blood: if the blood-pH value *drops*, the tissue-pH value *rises* (and vice versa). This gives us a kind of lever: it should be possible *indirectly* to *raise* an unhealthy acid-tissue-pH value by *lowering* the slightly alkaline blood-pH value. If there were a way to avoid the premature buffering of acid substances that are capable of lowering the blood-pH value, then consequently it would also be possible to reach the tissue (indirectly). This is, however, not possible with currently available acidic products.

However, nature provides a solution to this problem. Overacidification of tissue is prevented in a healthy organism by the dextrorotatory lactic acid that is constantly produced by movement and suitable nutrition. This, therefore, indicates that an input of optically dextrorotatory lactic acid is needed, as this acid cannot be buffered, and so acidifies the blood. My own investigations over many years have confirmed this point. This procedure may seem like a contradiction to the layman, in that tissue is to be *deacidified by administering an acid*. The paradox disappears, however, if all interrelations are kept in mind.

Acidification of the *blood* by means of dextrorotatory lactic acid lowers the blood-pH value until it and the tissue-pH value reach the same level. This takes precisely five weeks in cancer patients who are administered an appropriate dose of dextrorotatory lactic acid (thirty drops, three times daily). This has been confirmed time and again by my own measurements over many years of the blood-pH value. During the period from the first until approximately the fourth day in week 6, the acid substances will be discharged from the tissue into the blood, the pH value of which drops for a short time to very low values. The excretion of the pathological substances of the tissue via blood, liver, kidneys, and skin during this period is apparent from an extremely pungent and acid smell.

Overacidification of tissue can of course also be observed (or even be the norm) in individuals who are not afflicted by cancer. It is interesting to note that in such cases the pH value of tissue and blood becomes balanced after only two weeks, with administration of a lower daily dosage (three times twenty drops) of dextrorotatory lactic acid, or quite simply by strict fasting. The same effect can even be achieved by three weeks of a truly relaxing holiday and following roughly the above-described diet.

I am as yet unable to explain the reasons for the period of five (or two) weeks. However, the same physical and psychological symptoms occur after both these time intervals. Feeling generally unwell, the patient is irritable, aggressive, and depressed at the same time. At the height of this "changeover reaction," usually lasting for three days, the pH values of tissue and blood reach the same level, which the organism needs to rectify as quickly as possible, as otherwise the metabolism would cease to function.

> I recall the well-known test from my school days: a receptacle, which is split into two halves by a semipermeable membrane, has an acid solution on one side and an alkaline solution on the other. Immediately, an exchange of the liquids commences, until the same pH value is reached on both sides, and no further exchange takes place. This is what is happening in the metabolism.

The continued supply of dextrorotatory lactic acid finally ensures an unproblematic and physiological restitution and maintenance of a blood-pH value of 7.4 and a tissue-pH value above that figure. This will remove a critical precondition for continued growth of a tumor in a cancer patient, namely the acid environment. Kidneys and liver are now capable of carrying out their full detoxification functions, thereby, laying the foundations for a safe removal of subsequently occurring disintegration products of a malignant tumor. Finally, dextrorotatory lactic acid also causes the biological neutralization of the toxic, levorotatory lactic acid of the tumor into a nontoxic, racemic form. This is of utmost importance, as it removes the stimulus for an increase in the cell division rate.

Normalizing the acid-alkali balance also stimulates adrenaline production and improves its effectiveness, an equally important precondition for a healthy (aerobic) metabolism.

Restitution of Adrenaline Production

As adrenaline deficiency forms the core of this hypothesis on the formation of cancer, it must be endeavored to regenerate the *body's own production* of this hormone. This is best achieved with appropriate cell or organ preparations (Regeneresen therapy). The apparently obvious method, namely simply to inject adrenaline, must be rejected for two reasons.

First, no slow-release adrenaline preparation, remaining effective for longer than half an hour, is currently available (epinephrine preparations, used for stimulating circulation, are, therefore, unsuitable).

The second, and decisive, reason is that it would be futile to supply adrenaline, even if an appropriate preparation were available. Once this treatment was withdrawn, it would become apparent that the body's own adrenaline production had not been not reactivated but had instead become totally paralyzed comparable to the situation with adrenal cortex hormones (corticosteroids). A continuous, lifelong substitute supply of adrenaline is also inappropriate, because hardly any other hormone in the organism has to adapt itself to such an extent to continuously changing circumstances of physical and mental stress, muscle work, and resting. This type of flexibility over such a broad range of functions, as is the case with adrenaline, cannot be controlled "from outside."

It is, therefore, imperative that body-own production is stimulated. I have to admit that I am pursuing this rather pragmatically and in a seemingly complicated manner. The success over past decades of this therapy, based on a reasoned hypothesis, confirms, however, that it is appropriate for an illness that is, after all, not just a simple cold.

Enzymes, Vitamins

The disintegration process of tumor cells, which should be aided from the beginning by microwave therapy if possible, by injections which increase oxygen utilization, and by starving of malignant cells by means of the above-described diet, results not only in the formation of acid-waste products, but also of macromolecular protein particles, which are difficult to eliminate and often cause subfebrile temperatures. As this "fever" is rarely high enough to have a truly destructive effect on malignant cells, it only weakens the organism. (It must be borne in mind that such a symptom is often caused by albumin deficiency, which should then be remedied by one or several infusions).

The administration of combination preparations of digestion enzymes is recommended in order to facilitate the destruction of these particles. In any case, cancer patients often suffer from a deficiency of such enzymes. Oral application helps to stimulate the breaking down of food. Vitamin A, B, and C supplements are recommended, although opinions on supplements of B12 are divided. (Some published theses suggest that Vitamin B12 has a tumor-promoting effect. For this reason, a supplement of this vitamin should be avoided until conclusive, scientific clarification is available.) It is better to promote natural formation of vitamin B12 through detoxification of the intestinal flora and regulation of gastric secretion. The same is true for folic acid. Only following a subtotal gastrectomy (partial removal of the stomach) and after measurements have indicated a deficiency should these preparations be administered.

Sex Hormones

Sex hormones also can be used in the therapy of tumors.

The opinion, hitherto, was that administration of same-sex hormones is harmful in cases of *sex-hormone-dependent* new formations of tumors, even to the extent that attempts have been made to suppress the body's own production. However, the current opinion that the administration of *opposite*-sex hormones could contribute toward curing *sex-hormone-dependent* tumors is not one that I share, because in most cases, cancer patients are of an advanced age, when the body produces fewer rather than more hormones. It is also wrong to think that the organism will accept a supply of opposite-sex hormones without adverse reaction, because in addition to the *illusory suppression* of the body's own sex-hormone production (which is barely functioning or has ceased altogether), such an application will release a reaction in the anterior pituitary. *This will result in a strong stimulation of production of body-owned sex hormones and an even larger imbalance in the hormone system*—just the opposite of what it was supposed to achieve. Very often, patients undergoing this treatment register too high a testosterone level for men, and too high an oestrogen level for women.

The effect on the psyche through administration of opposite-sex hormones also needs to be taken into consideration. I have yet to meet a man, whatever his age, who would have been particularly happy to be a eunuch. This is dis-stress of the highest order, and the enormous strain this places on a partnership is of no help with the illness. Women have similar problems and suffer from depression and low self-esteem if they lose their womanhood.

Fortunately, present opinion is more in line with my own, namely that women patients with *sex-hormone-dependent* tumors should be given a low-dose replacement therapy of oestrogen alternating with progesterone, as examinations have shown that this can lead to a drastic improvement of both life expectancy and quality of life. Such a therapy does not only greatly enhance the mental state, but can also have the effect of an anabolic steroid so that it also serves to hold back the formation of skeletal metastases.

Such progressive thinking has, unfortunately, not yet taken place in terms of testosterone replacement therapy for men. I personally have never considered it harmful to allow patients at least the retention of the testosterone produced by their own body.

Same-sex sex hormones must of course not be supplied if the existing tumor proves to possess receptors for these, because this would indeed accelerate tumor growth.

Concluding Observations to the Therapy

Of course, not all tumors are curable with this therapy; but all tumors that are cured are either destroyed by inflammation (as previously described), or they simply disappear without major problems. It is possible for malignant tumors to become benign, operable tumors, although this is rare.

The therapy here introduced offers relatively great advantages to patients, because, the "changeover" reaction over three days excepted, they are not subjected to any stress. It is neither painful nor does it cause vomiting, loss of appetite, bleeding of the bladder, or other similar side effects that are well-known from aggressive therapies.

It does, however, require patience and time, which many patients and doctors find hard to provide. Listening to the patient and learning about his worries, even on a psychotherapeutic level, is time-consuming and is not covered by the health service. This is the more deplorable as the costs of primary therapies will be far greater in the long run and have a relatively uncertain outcome.

Open-minded contemporaries recognize that this therapy is based on a factual and plausible concept and, therefore, is far removed from being a trial-and-error method; treatment motive and treatment goal are always clear. Most of all, it is founded on a viewpoint that incorporates the *development history of cancer*, a viewpoint which is obviously alien to the normal approach of simply destroying tumor cells, however ambitious or perfected this may be. This therapy is not intended to be in opposition to known primary therapies but is intended to expand the available treatment methods with a successful outcome. If surgery, radiation, or chemotherapy become superfluous because the patient has effectively been cured—so much the better.

Outlook

There are two different aspects in the development of cancer: the phase up to the formation of the first cancer cells (precancer stage) and the phase of diagnosable-cancer illness. From this, it follows that it is possible

* to pursue a cancer therapy that is guided by the *emergence* of the cancer ; or
* to pursue a therapy that starts with the *existing cell aberrations* (which are relatively well researched nowadays).

Both the above are of course important, but it cannot be overlooked that at present all primary therapies still focus on the second aspect; and the causes for the malignant cell degeneration are consequently pushed into the background. UV light, tobacco smoke, and similar carcinogenic, environmental influences have been identified as potential risk factors, but a *more specific* interrelationship, which could fit with research into what takes place on a molecular level, has not yet been demonstrated. (The harmfulness of tobacco smoke is not disputed, but it is "only generally correct" as long as we do not know the reasons why not *every* smoker falls ill with cancer.)

The therapy here presented follows another path: at its core is the *development of the cancer*, or, more precisely, why natural defense mechanisms in the organism fail against carcinogenic influences while *still in the preliminary phase of the diagnosable cancer illness*. The basis is the idea that cancer develops over a longer period of time. When progress has been made in this direction, a therapy will first of all concentrate on the restitution of these natural defense mechanisms. I am of the opinion that this cancer-formation hypothesis offers a precise orientation for such a therapy. It has not been possible for me to provide conclusive theoretical support for the hypothesis in view of the high expenditure required for long-term scientific studies and similar. The hypothesis, therefore, has in places the character of *empirically* established *findings*, which need not detract from its value—on the contrary: a cured patient is happy about his recovered health, even without an "exact" explanation of all the biochemical processes, on a molecular level, which have led to both the illness and the cure. There is still the further task of underpinning both the hypothesis and the therapy by simultaneous laboratory tests, going beyond those that I have been conducting for years (i.e., in addition to the above-mentioned, customary laboratory tests, plotting progress curves of markers, measuring adrenaline levels, and of course carrying out scans).

Advances in science now make it possible with the aid of biochemical analyses to discover and measure the interrelationship between the hormones and the central and autonomous nervous systems, which to date had not been provable in the laboratory. A biochemical institute in London[28] has taken on board the cancer-formation hypothesis under discussion and as a first step has taken adrenaline measurements on one hundred cancer patients from outside my patient register; all their results support the hypothesis. So far, this confirms my own experiences and measurements; it has consequently heightened interest in the hypothesis. Further biochemical investigations brought to light highly interesting illness-specific changes in the neurotransmitters and their precursors, metabolites, derivates, and toxins in cancer patients. These findings could possibly lead to a change in the conception of cancer processes toward my hypothesis and consequently facilitate more accurate therapy progress monitoring. If the importance of such measuring parameters is recognized, they could in appropriately modified form become the basis for long-term studies of the cancer-formation phase and assist in explaining biochemically the interrelationships on a higher level (hormones, immune situation, acid-alkali household). This would at the same time shift the emphasis from looking at an individual cancer cell toward the whole system of "the living organism."

One thing is certain: processes such as we see in malignant aberrations will only happen in a biosystem that is out of balance—uncorrected gene mutations; chromosome ruptures; overactive oncogenes; and deactivated tumor-suppressor genes, inactive master genes, and aneuploidy.

Is It Possible to Protect Oneself Against Cancer?

Primary therapies attack tumors in a direct way, i.e., they attack the visible consequences of an illness, which has over a long period already developed through various stages. Surgery and radiation are palliative measures. Strictly speaking, they are only an attack on the symptoms, as for example the fear of a relapse after a successful operation clearly demonstrates. However, once the causes for the formation of cancer have been investigated and, as I believe, have been found, the therapy will follow another path—the path described in this book. People can of course also respond that they protect themselves against cancer by avoiding all the known triggers, but this is more easily said than done.

If the chain of events prior to the diagnosis of cancer is investigated, it is of course easy to blame present-day society for the *circumstances* leading to the formation of cancer discussed in this book. The choices open to the individual to avoid situations adversely affecting health are limited. We live in a society with a great many constraints. Hierarchical structures in the business world with their specific interpersonal and group-dynamic behavior patterns very often generate highly psychological stresses (pressures with regard to performance and competition, lack of recognition). Nerve-racking traffic jams in a carcinogenic-breathing environment occur ever more frequently; noise where holiday relaxation is needed, mad rush while eating *junk food*, irritation from the neighbour's lawnmower, the money-grabbing tax authorities, the shoddy car repair workshop, etc.—these more or less unavoidable stressors are permanent companions in modern life. There is hardly a route open for a healthy, physiological stress release—instead we are swamped with an overload of offers for leisure and entertainment. The question "*Is it possible to protect oneself against cancer?*" ultimately comes down to a way of life that corresponds with our nature that wants *not* to be overshadowed with permanent worry over doing something that is right and useful and avoiding doing something that is wrong and damaging. Unfortunately, we do not live in this state of "utopian innocence."

Our genetic inheritance, acquired through a lengthy period of evolution, must be brought into tune with today's civilization and culture that undergo more rapid and far-reaching changes than ever before in human history. It should be remembered that *Homo sapiens* is the result of a phylogenesis over millions of years and in the long process of evolution became equipped with characteristics that proved to be advantageous. However, in a modern highly technical civilization, which is subject to change in extremely short cycles, these characteristics are put to the test again. *Biological* evolution and *socio-cultural* evolution function as it were asynchronously. As a consequence, we now display behavior patterns, whether voluntarily or involuntarily, which "nature could not have anticipated," despite our being equipped with very flexible, inherent survival strategies. An organism equipped for movement with a sophisticated blood circulation; fine nerve connections; highly efficient joints, sinews, and muscles is in obvious conflict with the routine of sitting in a car in traffic chaos, breathing polluted air, then in an office chair, then back again having been subjected to all kinds of stress without an opportunity for abreaction, possibly ending the day slumped on a settee in front of the television.

I don't want to be misunderstood: cultural pessimism is not productive, and most people do not have the opportunity to escape from consumer-led society. We live in the modern world with all it offers, and our lives are made so much easier that all this has become indispensable to us. However, this has also generated many new problems, and we are on the path to endangering the foundations of our existence. As we make these changes, we must also accept our responsibilities, which become ever more far-reaching the more we contemplate them.

Almost everybody knows of the connection between CFCs (chlorofluorocarbons), the destruction of the ozone layer, and melanoma or that car exhaust fumes and emissions from the burning of fuel release carcinogens. If we change herbivores, such as cattle, into cannibals by thoughtlessly feeding them with their own reprocessed meat, nature gives us a dramatic lesson on our wrongdoing. Even if we are convinced that what we are doing is for the good, we can, nevertheless, create problems. We assist the immune system (e.g., by means of immunization and antibiotics) and, thus, discover that it acts in an incredibly sophisticated manner, because it is faced with an equally sophisticated opponent, which responds with dangerous mutations. Proof of this is given by the increasing resistance of many bacteria to synthetic antibiotics. This gives us an inkling of the challenges ahead of us.

> It seems that the humble honeybee is superior to us in this respect. Bees collect resin from plants, which they process into propolis and use in the construction of their hives. This provides an extremely effective, natural antibiotic having antifungal characteristics, against which bacteria (and even viruses) cannot develop a resistance. Bees coat the inside of their hives with a thin layer of propolis as protection against any possible infections. Even intruders killed by the bees, such as mice, are literally

embalmed with propolis to prevent the spread of infection. The beekeeper in his wisdom uses this antibiotic from nature's apothecary and surrounds the hive with mesh, which is immediately coated with propolis by the busy bees, which he can then scrape off. (This is not to romanticize nature, but it poses the question of who is superior to whom?)

It is clear that for a long time now we have been damaging nature—often irreversibly—whether out of ignorance or in full awareness, by upsetting the natural balance. There is much that is out of alignment, and we are paying the price for it; but fortunately, not everybody gets cancer immediately; however, the increase in tumorous illnesses cannot be overlooked. As a doctor, I do not wish to stray too far from my own specialized field and can and will, therefore, only give a rough outline of matters.

Does this mean that we are helplessly left to our fate and can only wait to see whether and when we will get "our cancer"? Of course not. There is a saying that everybody will ultimately get cancer if he lives long enough. How long is *long enough*? The same can be said for lightning strikes or any other fatal accidents. It is not about that. The number of young cancer patients is on the increase. Perhaps the lively centenarian who has never had cancer is lucky, but it was certainly not his ignorance about the formation of cancer that has protected him from this terrible illness. *More knowledge* about the interrelations does not harm; *less* knowledge can be fatal. This is one of the reasons why I have written this book.

I am, therefore, convinced that we have reason for optimism, because we are gaining an ever better understanding and are able to draw the appropriate conclusions from this. We have no other choice but to do so.

The quotation at the beginning is, therefore, of particular importance and is reiterated to conclude the circle:

> *He who knows the goal can decide.*
> *He who decides finds peace.*
> *He who finds peace is secure.*
> *He who is secure can reflect.*
> *He who reflects can improve.*

—Confucius

A Selection of Case Histories of Cured Patients

(Patients' names are not given in full to protect their anonymity. References to the present relate to the year 2003.)

Case 1

Gertrud S., born 1921. In April 1964, radium implant because of an inoperable cervical carcinoma, which had infiltrated into the left parametrium; good involution; in August 1966, relapse on pelvic wall. Husband was informed that patient's life expectancy would probably be until Christmas only. Bloody secretion from the crater, which had formed on the site of the radiated cervical carcinoma. Commencement of usual treatment; after three months, examination by gynecologist: complete involution of the infiltrate; right adnex clear; left adnex shows a scar the thickness of the little finger. Patient led a completely healthy life until 1982, when she died from a cause unrelated to cancer.

Case 2

Wolf Dieter L., born 1928. In August 1969, operation of a spindle-cell sarcoma of the skin over the sternum; three months after operative removal, relapse with metastases on axillary lymph nodes. Treatment as usual for about eight months, thereafter, recession of lymph node swelling and of relapse symptoms. To date, patient is alive and healthy.

Case 3

Christine K., born 1915. In 1968, radical surgery for carcinoma of the cervix. Patient consults me in March 1977 because of generalized bone metastases (confirmed histologically and by x-ray). Is treated by me for three months in the usual manner, and for a further seven months by her GP. Stops the treatment, after both clinical examination and x-rays show no sign of any residue of the formation of metastases. Patient continued her work as dressmaker and looked after her husband, who required day care. Patient was completely healthy until her death in 2001, aged eighty-six years.

Case 4

Rosel H., born 1913. In September 1978, after my discovering a huge ovarian tumor during a gynecological examination, operative removal of a partly cystoidal, partly solid-adnexal volleyball-sized tumor on the left, encapsulating the entire left urethra, peritoneal seeding, left-side pelvic-wall metastases. Histological diagnosis: papillary carcinoma, originating from left ovary, showing partial dysgerminoma-type differentiation. Husband of patient is informed that there is no chance of recovery or cure; given life expectancy of about three months. Commenced treatment with me in the usual manner; treatment course completely free of complications. The patient is healthy to date, attends to her housework, goes for walks, and has no ailments other than tinnitus.

Case 5

Adolf G., born 1958. Underwent surgery in August 1970 at the age of twelve, for a grade 2 astrocytoma of the cervical spinal cord between C2 and 3. Postoperative paresis of right arm. September 1971, operation because of relapse. November 1971, laminectomy for relief, as tumor had by then become inoperable. Patient comes into my care at this stage. He suffers from spastic paralysis of all extremities, is completely helpless, needs to be fed, and is incontinent. Surgeon anticipated life expectancy of three weeks. Treatment in the usual manner until March 1972; thereafter, patient can move his arms freely, feed and dress himself. Needs to use crutches because of remaining bilateral peroneal paresis. Subsequently, patient attends school and attains business qualification. In 1977, patient experiences renewed pain in the cervical spinal cord area and against my advice undergoes further surgery for a suspected neoplasmic relapse. The operation revealed, however, only a pea-size residuary neoplasm with rough-edged calcification. The operation left the patient paraplegic and wheelchair-bound, but to date, he is still healthy, living in Graz.

Case 6

Ursula R., born 1930. In July 1997, mammary carcinoma (adenocarcinoma) on left side. Undergoes neither operation nor other therapy before being treated by me in the usual manner. Patient has yearly checkups, is healthy to date, and goes frequently on adventure holidays with her partner.

Case 7

Swetlana M. W., born 1966. In June 1992, surgery for cystocarcinoma on right ovary; in April 1995, relapse—large tumor of the peritoneum, inoperable. Commencement of usual therapy, rapid shrinking of tumor. However, another year on, tumor is detectable by feel at nearly its former size but is now operable. Surgery reveals a completely encapsulated tumor; peritoneum is free of metastases. Histology of tumor: benign cystoma. Patient is healthy to date.

Case 8

Georg E., born 1928. In September 1983, diagnosis of carcinoma of the bladder. Treatment at University Clinic with repeat instillations of cytostatic agents. Commenced therapy with me after six further treatments for relapses. Five relapses while under my therapy; after several changes to natural therapies, patient has remained healthy since 1987.

Case 9

Manfred B., born 1935. In September 1971, diagnosis of testicular teratoma, followed by operation. Natural followup treatment in Zabel-Klinik, Bad Salzuflen. In August 1981, metastases on lymph nodes, surgery, then followup treatment with me. Patient is healthy to date and fathered children.

Case 10

Matthias H., born 1959. In 1997, surgical removal of disc epithelium carcinoma on tongue. In 1998, relapse with lymph-node metastases. Usual treatment with me; patient is healthy to date with no recurring symptoms.

Glossary

ACTH	adrenocorticotropic hormone, stimulates lypolysis together with adrenaline, noradrenalin, and glucagon
adrenaline	dioxyphenyl ethanol methylamine; also called epinephrine; hormone; formed in the cells of the adrenal gland and the sympathetic nerve cells; plays a central role in stress reaction
albumin	protein, water soluble, strongly hydrated, not precipitated by salt, carbohydrate free
aneuploidy	aberration of chromosomes in cancer cells, such as deviation in the number of chromosomes; or damaged chromosomes, for example missing, additional, or displaced DNA fragments
atheromatosis	degenerative changes on the inner layer of the arteries with atherosclerosis, a proliferation of fibrous tissues, leading to hardening and thickening of the inner wall of arteries
ATP	adenosine triphosphate, most important molecular vehicle of the cell for storing energy
atrophy	wasting of tissue through lack of nutrition of the tissue, or more generally disturbance of the metabolism processes, shifting the balance from building up to breaking down
atrophic	pertaining to the above symptoms
cachexia	wasting; atrophy of the organism as a result of serious disruption of all organ function; marked loss of weight, strength, and appetite; apathy and associated symptoms; also "tumor cachexia"
cytology	the study of the structure and functions of cells
cytostatic	having an inhibitory action on cell growth or cell division
DNA	deoxyribonucleic acid; molecular carrier of genetic information
ectoderm	outer germ layer of an embryo from which the central nervous system and sense organs are derived
ectodermal	pertaining to the ectoderm
ectopic	located outside its usual place

electrophoresis	motion of electrically charged particles in a fluid in a homogenous electric field
endometrium	smooth mucous membrane lining of the cavity of the uterus
erythrocytes	red blood corpuscles; cells lacking a nucleus with highly specialized anaerobic metabolism
erythropoietin	hormone produced in the kidneys, stimulating the formation of erythrocytes; released in response to decreased levels of oxygen in body tissue; for example, with certain types of anemia or at high altitude
fermentation	general term for various types of anaerobic metabolism with ATP as end product
γ-GT	Gamma-glutamyl transpeptidase; enzyme, increased levels of which indicate disintegration of carcinoma cells; is formed in kidneys, liver, and pancreas
globulins	collective term for a group of globular or rounded proteins, soluble in dilute salt solutions; most of the proteins in cells and body fluids belong to this group
granulocytes	type of white blood cells (leucocytes), acting as defense against infections
hormone	carrier or messenger, which can in minute quantities (micrograms) exercise a specific stimulatory physiological action on organs; examples are adrenaline, insulin, cortisone, glucagon, oestrogen, testosterone, etc.
hyaluronan	acidic, highly viscous, water-binding glycosaminoglycan; occurs in the organism as base substance of connective tissue, synovial fluid, the umbilical cord, skin, and the vitreous humour; also in haemolytic streptococci; is broken down by hyaluronidase; regulates cell permeability; lubricates; protective agent against infectious germs
hyaluronidase	enzyme, splits, i.e., depolymerizes hyaluronic acid; increases permeability of connective and supportive tissues and facilitates fluid exchange between tissues and capillary system; aids dispersion of foreign substances; promotes absorption of infusions and injections; the effect is restricted by adrenaline, for example
hypertonia	a state of abnormally high tension or pressure
hypothalamus	part of the midbrain lying below the thalamus; acts as central regulatory organ of autonomous functions, such as absorption of nutrition and water, circulation, body temperature, sex, sleep
insulin	hormone, regulates the metabolism of carbohydrates together with glucagon, adrenaline, and somatostatin; formed in the pancreas, lowers blood sugar level, and plays a crucial role in diabetes
invertose	optically levorotatory mixture of equal parts of glucose and fructose, main constituent of honey

lactose	sugar found in milk
LATS	long-acting thyroid stimulator; presence indicates hyperthyroidism
LDH	lactate dehydrogenase, enzyme that catalyzes the formation and removal of lactate
lipolysis	breaking down of fat by mobilizing body fat
lipolytic	pertaining to the breaking down of fat
luteinising hormone	a gonadotrophic hormone that is secreted by the anterior pituitary; stimulates ovulation in females and stimulates androgen release in males
lysosome	a membrane-bound organelle in the cytoplasm of most cells containing various hydrolytic enzymes that function in intracellular digestion of nucleic acids, glycogen, proteins, glycosaminoglycans, lipids
macrophage	long-living, nomadic cells stemming from the blood monocytes; key function in humoral immune response
metabolism	sum total of the chemical processes that occur in living organisms, producing energy, growth, eliminating waste, etc.
metastasis	the spreading of a disease organism, especially cancer cells, from one part of the body to another
mitochondria	organelles intimately concerned in certain enzyme processes within the cell, e.g., cell respiration; center of ATP production by means of phosphorylation
mycoplasma	pathogenic single-cell organisms lacking a cell wall
necrosis	death of one or more cells within a localized area, while still part of the living body; serious consequence of a disruption in the metabolism, e.g., oxygen deficiency
noradrenalin	also called norepinephrine; hormone, having similar properties to adrenaline and differing in structure by one methyl group only
paraneoplastic	having a remote effect on a humoral path, originating from a tumor or its metastases; paraneoplastically formed hormones and peptides with hormonelike effect cause metabolic or degenerative changes at the responding organs. For example: thrombosis with cancer of the pancreas; hypercalcemia with genito-urinary cancers.
pH value	indicates the level of acidity or alkalinity on a scale of 0 to 14; water having the median value of 7
phosphatase	any of a group of enzymes which hydrolyze orthophosphoric esters to phosphoric acid and alcohol; alkaline phosphatases (AP) are distributed in cells and body fluids
phosphorylation	the addition of phosphate to an organic compound; the enzymatic conversion of carbohydrates into their phosphoric esters in metabolic processes
pituitary gland	also known as the hypophysis, roughly the size of a hazelnut, encapsulated by connective tissue, situated at the base of the midbrain

propolis	natural antibiotic; resinous substance collected by bees from buds of trees and processed in their hives
racemic	pertaining to a mixture of dextrorotatory and levorotatory isomers in such proportions that it has no optical effect
retroviruses	RNA viruses having the characteristic of infiltrating their genes into the DNA-cell nucleus of an infected host cell, where they may remain undetected over a long period of time (years), but ultimately they change the cell and bring about its destruction
serotonin	hormone particularly found in brain and intestinal tissue, blood platelets, and mast cells; acts as neurotransmitter
sorbitol	sweetener used as a sugar substitute for diabetics
sympathicotonia	permanent shift from autonomic balance in favor of the sympathetic nervous system, i.e., increased stimulation of the sympathetic system
thrombocytes	cells with essential function in blood clotting; have no nucleus; broken down in the spleen
thyrotropic	pertaining to the stimulation of the thyroid
ulcer	localized destruction of the surface of the skin or mucous membrane; a result of an infection or of an illness in general; usually heals leaving a scar after the dead tissue has been discarded
vagotonia	also called parasympathicotonia; permanent shift from the autonomic balance to the parasympathetic nervous system, i.e., increased stimulation of parasympathetic system

References

(A few references relate to personal correspondence, discussions, or talks, which can no longer be dated accurately.)

1) Francis Crick (British) together with James Watson (American), discovered in Cambridge on 28 February 1953 the double-helix structure of DNA. Twenty years later Watson published his now famous book *The Double Helix*.
2) As per Ernst Mayr: Das ist Biologie, Die Wissenschaft des Lebens, Spektrum Akad. Verlag 2000. The main work is *Systematics and the Origin of Species*, 1942. Mayr is recognized worldwide as the most important evolutionary biologist of our time. Fundamental contributions to connecting Darwinism with modern genetics. Harvard University, where he was a lecturer for many years, named the library of the department of comparative zoology the "Ernst-Mayr Library"—a rare honor.
3) As per A. Maier, historian, 1938.
4) cf. Christoph A. Klein, Institute for Immunology, Munich University, 2003.
5) cf. A. von Metzler and C. Nitsch, Max Planck Institute for Brain Research, Frankfurt, Naturwissenschaften 10, 1985.
6) As per Manfred Eigen, Stufen zum Leben, die frühe Evolution im Visier der Molekularbiologie, Piper, Munich Zurich, 1987.
7) cf. also William J. Schopf, Die Evolution der ersten Zellen, Spektrum der Wissenschaften, Evolution, 1988.
8) cf. Seeger.
9) cf. Sir Gustav J. V. Nossal, Das Immunsystem. The exploration of the defense system, its role in life, sickness, and death, establishes a scientific framework for understanding the functioning of the organism as a whole, Spektrum der Wissenschaft, Spezial 2, 1997.
10) See also Charles A. Janeway, Paul Travers, Mark Walport, Mark Shlomchik, Immunology, Spektrum-Verlag, Heidelberg Berlin, 2002.

11) cf. H. P. Kluza, A. J. Moritz, Münchener Medizinische Wochenschrift, 1985.
12) cf. Rosenberg, online issue of *Science Magazine*, September, 2002.
13) cf. Berger, Deutsches Krebsforschungs-Institut (German Cancer Research Institute) Heidelberg, 1982.
14) cf. Labhardt, Klinik der Inneren Sekretion, 2nd edition, 1971.
15) cf. *German Medical Weekly Journal*, 50/1982.
16) cf. Berger, Deutsches Krebsforschungs-Institut (German Cancer Research Institute) Heidelberg, Selecta, 1982.
17) cf. Weiß, Leipzig, Lecture at Cancer Convention in Baden-Baden, 1976.
18) cf. Frederic Vester, Phänomen Streß: where is its origin; why is it essential for life; what causes its degeneration? Deutscher Taschenbuch Verlag, Munich, 2003.
19) cf. Tausk.
20) cf. Schulze, Marburg.
21) cf. Aschoff, Scylway, Seeger.
22) cf. Warburg, Seeger.
23) See also Karin Ahlberg in *The Lancet*, June 2003.
24) See *Frankfurter Allgemeine*, daily newspaper, 17 June 2003.
25) See Hans Selye, Streß-mein Leben, Kindler Verlag, Munich, 1979.
26) cf. Jäger in Münchener Medizinische Wochenschrift No. 125, 1983.
27) See also C. G. Jung, Psychological Types, 1921.
28) cf. O. Galkina, Neurotech Institute, London, 2003.

Index

A

ACTH (adrenal cortical hormones), 43
adaptive immunity, 35
adrenaline, 26, 29, 31
    deficiency, 26, 31, 33, 66
AIDS (acquired immune deficiency syndrome), 21
allergy stage, 60

B

biology
    holism, 16
    reductionism, 16, 25
blood-oxygen supply, 31, 34
breast cancer, 19
B cells (B lymphocytes), 36

C

calcitonin, 47
cancer, 21
    acid-alkali imbalance, 48, 65
    cell-based degeneration, 18
    diagnosis, 18
    formation process, 45
    hereditary traits, 56
    medical recommendations, 49, 63
    personality types, 56
    possible causes, 21, 23, 37
    prevention, 17
    primary therapies, 15, 22
    recommended diet, 62
    tests on animals, 28
    treatment, 69
        enzymes and vitamins, 67
        hormones, 68
        side effects, 69
    tumor formation, 59
    viruses leading to, 23
        cells, 22
        genes, 24
cancer-patient cases, 74
Cannons stress theory, 51
cells, 20, 22
    aerobic metabolism, 32
    anaerobic metabolism, 32
    sugar, 31
cellular immunity, 36
chemotherapy, 37
chromaffin system, 29
congenital immunity, 35

D

dextrorotatory lactic acid, 34, 49, 65
    cancer treatment, 66
diabetes, 40, 44

E

eukaryotes, 32
extroverts, 57

F

fermentation, 33

G

general adaptation syndrome. *See* Selye syndrome
glucagon, 44
glucocorticoids. *See* adrenal cortical hormones
glycogen, 33, 47

H

Hippocrates, 56
hormones, 30, 46
  adrenaline, 30
  importance, 42
  insulin, 39
humoral immunity, 36
hypergy, 60

I

immune response, 35
immune system, 35, 72
  protection, 37
immune therapies, 37
infection, 35
insulin, 26, 31
  possible cancer cause, 40
  uses, 40
introverts, 57

J

Janke stress model, 52

L

Lazarus stress model, 52
levorotatory lactic acid, 33

M

malignant tumor, 23
metabolism, 33
multipurpose principle, 42

N

noradrenaline, 26, 31
normergy, 59

O

oncogenes, 24, 40

P

Pasteur, Louis, 33
pathogens, 35
patients, 27
pH value, 48, 65
prokaryotes, 32
psycho drugs, 28

S

Schwann, Theodor, 20
scientific revolution, 16
Selye, Hans, 51
Selyes stress theory, 52
Selye syndrome, 53
STH (somatotropic hormone), 44
stress, 26, 29, 51
  causes, 53
  dis-stress, 52
  eustress, 52
sympathicotonic personality, 57
sympathomimetic drugs, 28

T

thyroid hormones, 43
tumor, 18, 24, 37, 38, 47
tumor-suppressor genes, 24
T cells (T lymphocytes), 36

V

vagotonic personality, 56
vitalism, 16
vitamin B12, 67

www.ingramcontent.com/pod-product-compliance
Lightning Source LLC
Chambersburg PA
CBHW021003180526
45163CB00005B/1880